LIPP
of NU

Series

ECG
INTERPRETATION

◆

 Wolters Kluwer | Lippincott Williams & Wilkins
Health

Philadelphia • Baltimore • New York • London
Buenos Aires • Hong Kong • Sydney • Tokyo

STAFF

Executive Publisher
Judith A. Schilling McCann, RN, MSN

Editorial Director
H. Nancy Holmes

Clinical Director
Joan M. Robinson, RN, MSN

Art Director
Mary Ludwicki

Editorial Project Manager
Sean Webb

Editors
Jennifer Lynn Kowalak,
Carol Turkington

Clinical Editor
Elizabethe Westgard, RN, MSN

Copy Editors
Kimberly Bilotta, Laura Healy,
Marna Poole, Jenifer Walker

Designers
Marsha Biderman, Jan Greenberg,
Joseph John Clark

Digital Composition Services
Diane Paluba (manager),
Joyce Rossi Biletz, Donna S. Morris

Manufacturing
Beth J. Welsh

Editorial Assistants
Megan L. Aldinger, Karen J. Kirk,
Linda K. Ruhf

Indexer
Deborah Tourtlotte

The clinical treatments described and recommended in this publication are based on research and consultation with nursing, medical, and legal authorities. To the best of our knowledge, these procedures reflect currently accepted practice. Nevertheless, they can't be considered absolute and universal recommendations. For individual applications, all recommendations must be considered in light of the patient's clinical condition and, before administration of new or infrequently used drugs, in light of the latest package-insert information. The authors and publisher disclaim any responsibility for any adverse effects resulting from the suggested procedures, from any undetected errors, or from the reader's misunderstanding of the text.

LMNPECG010507

**Library of Congress
Cataloging-in-Publication Data**

ECG interpretation.
        p. ; cm. — (Lippincott manual of nursing practice series)
    Includes bibliographical references.
    1. Electrocardiography—Handbooks, manuals, etc. 2. Heart—Diseases—Nursing—Handbooks, manuals, etc. I. Series.
    [DNLM: 1. Electrocardiography—nursing—Handbooks. WY 49 E17 2008]
    RC683.5.E5E252 2008
    616.1'207547—dc22
ISBN-13: 978-0-7817-7741-4 (alk. paper)
ISBN-10: 0-7817-7741-0 (alk. paper) 2007005855

CONTENTS

◆

CONTRIBUTORS AND CONSULTANTS

Gary J. Arnold, MD
Associate Professor
College of Nursing and Allied Health
    Professions
University of Louisiana at Lafayette

**Cheryl A. Bean, APRN, BC, DSN, ANP,
    AOCN**
Associate Professor/Adult Nurse Practitioner
Indiana University School of Nursing
Indianapolis

Mary Ann Boucher, APRN, BC, ND
Assistant Professor of Nursing
University of Massachusetts Dartmouth

Peggy Bozarth, RN, MSN
Professor
Hopkinsville (Ky.) Community College

Janie Choate, PA-C, MAT, BS, BA
Adjunct Faculty
University of the Sciences
Philadelphia

Laura M. Criddle, RN, MS, CCNS, CEN
Doctoral Student
Oregon Health & Science University
Portland

Diane Dixon, PA-C, MA, MMSc
Assistant Professor and Academic Coordinator
University of South Alabama
Department of Physician Assistant Studies
Mobile

Shirley Lyon Garcia, RN, BSN
Nursing Program Director, PNE
McDowell Technical Community College
Marion, N.C.

Charla K. Hollin, RN, BSN
Nursing Program Director
Rich Mountain Community College
Mena, Ark.

**Shelley Yerger Huffstutler, RN, DSN,
    CFNP, GNP**
Associate Professor and Director, FNP Program
University of Alabama at Birmingham
    School of Nursing

Mary T. Kowalski, RN, BA, MSN
*Director Vocational Nursing and Health Career
    Programs*
Cerro Coso Community College
Ridgecrest, Calif.

Grace G. Lewis, RN, MS, BC
Assistant Professor of Nursing
Georgia Baptist College of Nursing of
    Mercer University
Atlanta

Patricia J. McBride, RN, MSN, CIC
Infection Control Manager
Bryn Mawr (Pa.) Hospital

Cynthia A. Prows, RN, MSN, CNS
Clinical Nurse Specialist
Children's Hospital Medical Center
Cincinnati

Betty E. Sims, RN, MSN
Nurse Consultant
Board of Nurse Examiners
Austin, Tex.
Adjunct Instructor
St. Philip's College
San Antonio, Tex.

Sheryl Thomas, RN, MSN
Nurse Instructor
Wayne County Community College
Detroit

Dan Vetrosky, PA-C, MEd, PhD(c)
Assistant Professor
University of South Alabama
Mobile

Colleen R. Walsh, RN, MSN, ACNP-BC,
  CS, ONC
Faculty, Graduate Nursing
University of Southern Indiana School of
    Nursing & Health Professions
Evansville

PART 1

◆

Reviewing fundamentals

CARDIAC ANATOMY AND PHYSIOLOGY

Correct electrocardiogram (ECG) interpretation is a challenge for any practitioner. With a good understanding of ECGs, you'll be better able to provide expert care to your patients. For example, when you're caring for a patient with an arrhythmia or a myocardial infarction, an ECG waveform can help you quickly assess his condition and begin lifesaving interventions.

To build ECG skills, start with the basics covered in this chapter—an overview of the heart's anatomy and physiology.

Cardiac anatomy

The heart is a hollow muscular organ that works like a mechanical pump. It delivers oxygenated blood to the body through the arteries. When blood returns through the veins, the heart pumps it to the lungs to be reoxygenated. In this section you'll find descriptions of the location and structure of the heart, how blood flows through the heart, and the coronary blood supply.

LOCATION AND STRUCTURE

The heart lies at an angle in the chest, behind the sternum in the mediastinal cavity, or mediastinum. It's located between the lungs, in front of the spine. The top of the heart, called the base, lies just below the second rib. The bottom of the heart, called the apex, tilts forward and down toward the left side of the body and rests on the diaphragm. (See *The heart's location,* page 4.)

An infant's heart is positioned more horizontally in the chest cavity than an adult's heart. As a result, the apex is at the fourth intercostal space. Until age 4, the apical impulse is to the left of the midclavicular line. By age 7, the child's heart is located in the adult position.

The heart varies in size, depending on a person's body size, but it's roughly 5" (12 cm) long and 3¼" (8 cm) wide, or about the size of a fist. The heart's weight, typically 9 to 12 oz (255 to 340 g), varies depending on the person's size, age, sex, and athletic conditioning. An athlete's heart usually weighs more than average, and an elderly person's heart usually weighs less than average.

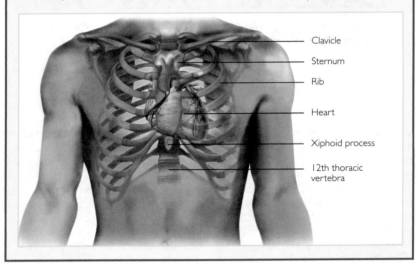
As a person ages, his heart usually becomes slightly smaller and loses its strength and efficiency. People with hypertension may experience a moderate increase in left ventricular wall thickness. As the heart ages, the myocardium becomes more easily irritated and extrasystoles may occur, along with sinus arrhythmias and sinus bradycardias. In addition, increased fibrous tissue infiltrates the sinoatrial (SA) node and internodal atrial tracts, which may cause atrial fibrillation and flutter.

By age 70, cardiac output at rest has diminished by 30% to 35% in many people.

Heart wall
The heart wall is made up of three layers:

- the epicardium (the outermost layer) is made of squamous epithelial cells overlying connective tissue
- the myocardium (the middle and thickest layer) is the largest portion of the heart's wall and contracts with each heartbeat
- the endocardium (the heart wall's innermost layer) consists of a thin layer of endothelial tissue that lines the heart valves and chambers. (See *Layers of the heart wall*.)

Pericardium
The pericardium is a fluid-filled sac that envelops the heart and acts as a tough, protective covering. It consists of the fibrous pericardium and the serous pericardium. The fibrous pericardium is made of tough, white tissue, which fits loosely around the heart and protects it. The serous

LAYERS OF THE HEART WALL

This cross-section of the heart wall shows its various layers.

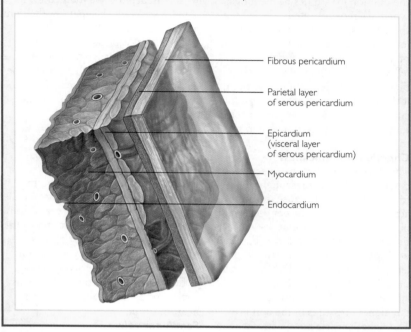

Fibrous pericardium

Parietal layer
of serous pericardium

Epicardium
(visceral layer
of serous pericardium)

Myocardium

Endocardium

pericardium is the thin, smooth, inner portion, and includes two layers: the *parietal layer,* which lines the inside of the fibrous pericardium, and the *visceral layer,* which adheres to the surface of the heart.

The pericardial space separates the visceral and parietal layers and contains 10 to 30 ml of thin, clear pericardial fluid that lubricates the two surfaces and cushions the heart.

Heart chambers
The heart contains four chambers—two atria and two ventricles.
Atria
The right atrium lies in front of and to the right of the smaller, thicker-walled left atrium. An interatrial septum sepa-

rates the two chambers and helps them contract. The right and left atria serve as volume reservoirs for blood being sent into the ventricles. The right atrium receives deoxygenated blood returning from the body through the inferior and superior venae cavae and from the heart through the coronary sinus. The left atrium receives oxygenated blood from the lungs through the four pulmonary veins. Contraction of the atria forces blood into the ventricles.
Ventricles
The right and left ventricles serve as the pumping chambers of the heart. The right ventricle lies behind the sternum and forms the largest part of the heart's sternocostal surface and

inferior border. The right ventricle receives deoxygenated blood from the right atrium and pumps it through the pulmonary arteries to the lungs, where it's reoxygenated. The left ventricle forms the heart's apex, most of its left border, and most of its posterior and diaphragmatic surfaces. The left ventricle receives oxygenated blood from the left atrium and pumps it through the aorta into the systemic circulation. The interventricular septum separates the ventricles and helps them pump.

Chamber wall thickness

The thickness of a chamber's walls is determined by the pressure needed to eject its blood. Because the atria act as reservoirs for the ventricles and pump the blood a shorter distance, their walls are much thinner than the walls of the ventricles. Likewise, the left ventricle has a much thicker wall than the right ventricle because the left ventricle pumps blood against the higher pressures in the aorta. The right ventricle pumps blood against the lower pressures in the pulmonary circulation.

Heart valves

The heart contains four valves—two atrioventricular (AV) valves (tricuspid and mitral) and two semilunar valves (aortic and pulmonic). Each valve consists of cusps, or leaflets, that open and close in response to pressure changes within the chambers they connect. The primary function of the valves is to keep blood flowing forward through the heart. When the valves close, they prevent backflow, or regurgitation, of blood between chambers. The sounds of the valves closing is what causes the heart sounds.

AV valves

The two AV valves located between the atria and ventricles are:
- the tricuspid valve (named for its three cusps), which separates the right atrium from the right ventricle
- the mitral valve (sometimes referred to as the bicuspid valve because of its two cusps), which separates the left atrium from the left ventricle.

The closing AV valves make the S_1—the first heart sound.

The cusps of these valves are anchored to the papillary muscles of the ventricles by small tendinous cords called chordae tendineae. During ventricular contraction, the papillary muscles and chordae tendineae work together to prevent the cusps from bulging backward into the atria. Disruption of either of these structures may prevent valves from closing completely, allowing blood to flow backward into the atria. This backward blood flow may cause a heart murmur.

Semilunar valves

The semilunar valves, so called because their three cusps resemble half moons, are:
- the pulmonic valve, located where the pulmonary artery meets the right ventricle; this valve permits blood to flow from the right ventricle to the pulmonary artery and prevents backflow into the right ventricle
- the aortic valve, located where the left ventricle meets the aorta; this valve allows blood to flow from the left ventricle to the aorta and prevents blood backflow into the left ventricle.

Increased pressure within the ventricles during ventricular systole causes the pulmonic and aortic valves to open, ejecting blood into the pulmonary and systemic circulation. Loss of pressure as the ventricular

INSIDE A NORMAL HEART

This cross-section shows the internal structure of a normal heart.

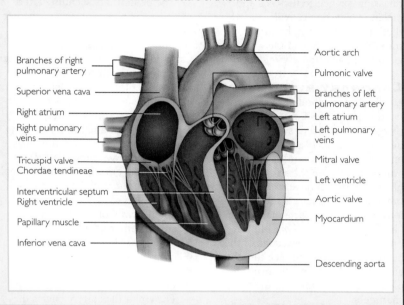

Branches of right pulmonary artery

Superior vena cava

Right atrium

Right pulmonary veins

Tricuspid valve
Chordae tendineae

Interventricular septum
Right ventricle

Papillary muscle

Inferior vena cava

Aortic arch

Pulmonic valve

Branches of left pulmonary artery

Left atrium

Left pulmonary veins

Mitral valve

Left ventricle

Aortic valve

Myocardium

Descending aorta

chambers empty causes the valves to close. The closing of the semilunar valves makes the S_2, or the second heart sound.

BLOOD FLOW THROUGH THE HEART

Learning how blood flows through the heart is critical for understanding the overall functions of the heart and how changes in electrical activity affect peripheral blood flow. It's also important to remember that right and left heart events occur at the same time. (See *Inside a normal heart.*)

Deoxygenated blood from the body returns to the heart through the inferior vena cava, superior vena cava, and coronary sinus and empties into the right atrium. The increasing volume of blood in the right atrium

raises the pressure in that chamber above the pressure in the right ventricle. Then, the tricuspid valve opens, allowing blood to flow into the right ventricle.

The right ventricle pumps blood through the pulmonic valve into the pulmonary arteries and lungs, where oxygen is picked up and excess carbon dioxide is released. From the lungs, the oxygenated blood flows through the pulmonary veins and into the left atrium. This completes the circuit called pulmonary circulation.

As the volume of blood in the left atrium increases, the pressure in the left atrium exceeds the pressure in the left ventricle. The mitral valve opens, allowing blood to flow into the left ventricle. The ventricle contracts and ejects the blood through the aortic valve into the aorta. The blood is distributed throughout the body, releasing oxygen to the cells and picking up carbon dioxide. Blood then returns to the right atrium through the veins, completing a circuit called systemic circulation.

CORONARY BLOOD SUPPLY

Like brain and all other organs, the heart needs an adequate supply of oxygenated blood to survive. The heart receives its blood supply almost entirely through the main coronary arteries that lie on the surface of the heart, and which have smaller arterial branches that penetrate the surface into the cardiac muscle mass. (See *Vessels that supply the heart*.) In fact, only a very small percentage of the heart's endocardial surface can obtain enough nutrition directly from the blood that flows through the cardiac chambers.

Understanding coronary blood flow can help you provide better care for a patient with coronary artery disease because you'll be able to predict which areas of the heart would be affected by narrowing or an occlusion in a particular coronary artery.

Coronary arteries

The left main and right coronary arteries ascend from the coronary ostia, small orifices located just above the aortic valve cusps. The right coronary artery fills the groove between the atria and ventricles, becoming the acute marginal artery and ending as the posterior descending artery. The right coronary artery supplies blood to the:
- right atrium
- right ventricle

- inferior wall of the left ventricle
- SA node in about 50% of people
- AV node in 90% of people.

The posterior descending artery supplies the posterior wall of the left ventricle in about 85% of people.

The left main coronary artery varies in length from a few millimeters to a few centimeters. It splits into two major branches, the left anterior descending (also known as the interventricular) and the left circumflex arteries. The left anterior descending artery runs down the anterior surface of the heart toward the apex. This artery and its branches—the diagonal arteries and the septal perforators—supply blood to the:
- anterior wall of the left ventricle
- anterior interventricular septum
- bundle of His
- right bundle branch
- anterior fasciculus of the left bundle branch.

The circumflex artery circles the left ventricle, ending on its posterior surface. The obtuse marginal artery arises from the circumflex artery. The circumflex artery provides oxygenated blood to the:
- lateral wall of the left ventricle
- left atrium
- posterior wall of the left ventricle in 10% of people
- posterior fasciculus of the left bundle branch
- SA node in about 50% of people
- AV node in about 10% of people.

In most people, the right coronary artery is the dominant vessel, meaning the right coronary artery supplies the posterior wall via the posterior descending artery. This is described as right coronary dominance or a dominant right coronary artery. Likewise, when the left coronary artery supplies

VESSELS THAT SUPPLY THE HEART

Coronary circulation involves the arterial system of blood vessels, which supplies oxygenated blood to the heart, and the venous system, which removes oxygen-depleted blood from the heart.

Anterior view

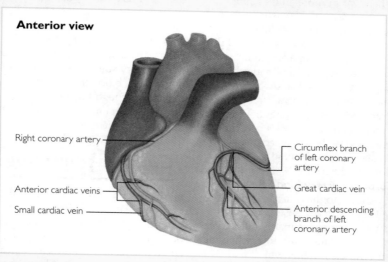

Right coronary artery

Anterior cardiac veins

Small cardiac vein

Circumflex branch of left coronary artery

Great cardiac vein

Anterior descending branch of left coronary artery

Posterior view

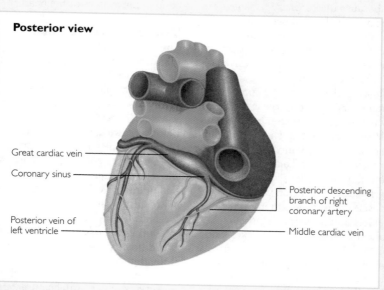

Great cardiac vein

Coronary sinus

Posterior vein of left ventricle

Posterior descending branch of right coronary artery

Middle cardiac vein

the posterior wall via the posterior descending artery, the terms *left coronary dominance* or *dominant left coronary artery* are used.

Collateral circulation

When two or more arteries supply the same region, they usually connect through anastomoses—junctions that provide alternate routes of blood flow. This network of smaller arteries, called collateral circulation, provides blood to capillaries that directly feed the heart muscle. Collateral circulation often becomes so strong that even if major coronary arteries become narrowed with plaque, collateral circulation can continue to supply blood to the heart.

Coronary artery blood flow

In contrast to the other vascular beds in the body, the heart receives its blood supply primarily during ventricular relaxing or diastole, when the left ventricle is filling with blood. This is because the coronary ostia lie near the aortic valve and become partially occluded when the aortic valve opens during ventricular contracting or systole. When the aortic valve closes, the ostia are unobstructed, allowing blood to fill the coronary arteries. Because diastole is the time when the coronary arteries receive the blood, anything that shortens diastole, such as periods of increased heart rate or tachycardia, will also decrease coronary blood flow.

In addition, the left ventricular muscle compresses intramuscular vessels during systole. During diastole, the cardiac muscle relaxes, and bloodflow through the left ventricular capillaries is no longer obstructed.

Cardiac veins

Just as other parts of the body do, the heart has its own veins, which remove oxygen-depleted blood from the myocardium. About 75% of the total coronary venous blood flow leaves the left ventricle by way of the coronary sinus, an enlarged vessel that returns blood to the right atrium. Most of the venous blood from the right ventricle flows directly into the right atrium through the small anterior cardiac veins, not by way of the coronary sinus. A small amount of coronary blood flows back into the heart through the thebesian veins, tiny veins that empty directly into all chambers of the heart.

Cardiac physiology

In this section you'll find descriptions of the cardiac cycle, cardiac output, autonomic innervation, transmission of electrical impulses, depolarization and repolarization, and the electrical conduction system of the heart.

THE CARDIAC CYCLE

The cardiac cycle includes events that occur from the beginning of one heartbeat to the beginning of the next. The cardiac cycle consists of ventricular diastole (relaxing) and ventricular systole (contracting). During ventricular diastole, blood flows from the atria through the open tricuspid and mitral valves into the relaxed ventricles. The aortic and pulmonic valves close during ventricular diastole. (See *Phases of the cardiac cycle.*)

During diastole, about 75% of the blood flows passively from the atria through the open tricuspid and mitral valves and into the ventricles before the atria contract. Atrial contraction, or atrial kick, contributes another 25% to ventricular filling. Loss of

PHASES OF THE CARDIAC CYCLE

The cardiac cycle consists of these phases:

1. Isovolumetric ventricular contraction—In response to ventricular depolarization, tension in the ventricles increases. The rise in pressure within the ventricles leads to closure of the mitral and tricuspid valves. The pulmonic and aortic valves stay closed during the entire phase.
2. Ventricular ejection—When ventricular pressure exceeds aortic and pulmonary artery pressures, the aortic and pulmonic valves open and the ventricles eject blood.
3. Isovolumetric relaxation—When ventricular pressure falls below the pressures in the aorta and pulmonary artery, the aortic and pulmonic valves close. All valves are closed during this phase. Atrial diastole occurs as blood fills the atria.
4. Ventricular filling—When atrial pressure exceeds ventricular pressure, the mitral and tricuspid valves open. Blood then flows passively into the ventricles. About 70% of ventricular filling takes place during this phase.
5. Atrial systole—Known as the atrial kick, atrial systole (coinciding with late ventricular diastole) supplies the ventricles with the remaining 30% of the blood for each heartbeat.

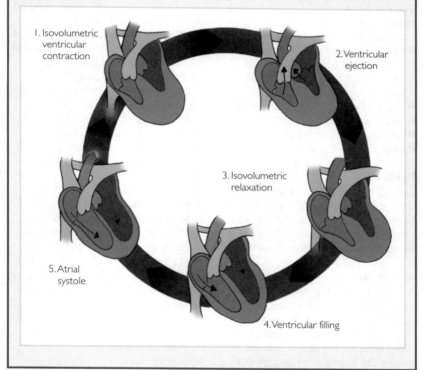

1. Isovolumetric ventricular contraction

2. Ventricular ejection

3. Isovolumetric relaxation

5. Atrial systole

4. Ventricular filling

effective atrial contraction occurs in some arrhythmias, such as atrial fibrillation, which leads to reduced cardiac output.

During ventricular systole, the mitral and tricuspid valves are closed as the relaxed atria fill with blood. As ventricular pressure rises, the aortic and pulmonic valves open. The ventricles contract and eject blood into the pulmonic and systemic circulation.

CARDIAC OUTPUT

Cardiac output is the amount of blood the left ventricle pumps into the aorta per minute. It's calculated by multiplying the heart rate times the stroke volume. Stroke volume is the amount of blood ejected with each ventricular contraction, and is usually about 70 ml.

Normal cardiac output is 4 to 8 L per minute, depending on body size. The heart pumps only as much blood as the body requires, based on metabolic requirements. During exercise, for example, the heart increases cardiac output accordingly.

Three factors determine stroke volume:
- preload
- afterload
- myocardial contractility. (See *Preload and afterload*.)

Preload

Preload is the degree of stretch or tension on the muscle fibers when they begin to contract. It's usually considered to be the end-diastolic pressure when the ventricle has become filled.

Afterload

Afterload is the load or amount of pressure the left ventricle must work against to eject blood during systole, and corresponds to the systolic pressure—the stronger this resistance, the greater the heart's workload. Afterload is also called *systemic vascular resistance*.

Myocardial contractility

The degree of muscle fiber stretch at the end of diastole determines the ventricle's ability to contract (also

called contractility). The more the muscle fibers stretch during ventricular filling, up to the optimal length, the more forceful the contraction.

AUTONOMIC INNERVATION

The two branches of the autonomic nervous system—the sympathetic (or adrenergic) and the parasympathetic (or cholinergic)—abundantly supply the heart. Sympathetic fibers innervate all the areas of the heart, while parasympathetic fibers primarily innervate the SA and AV nodes.

Sympathetic nerve stimulation triggers the release of norepinephrine, which boosts the heart rate, by increasing SA-node discharge, accelerating AV-node–conduction time, and increasing the force of myocardial contraction and cardiac output.

Parasympathetic (vagal) stimulation triggers the release of acetylcholine, which produces the opposite effects. The rate of SA-node discharge drops, which slows conduction through the AV node, heart rate, and cardiac output.

TRANSMISSION OF ELECTRICAL IMPULSES

For the heart to contract and pump blood to the rest of the body, an electrical stimulus is needed. Generation and transmission of electrical impulses depend on these four key characteristics of cardiac cells:
- automaticity
- conductivity
- contractility
- excitability.

Automaticity refers to a cell's ability to spontaneously initiate an electrical impulse. Pacemaker cells usually possess this ability. Excitability results from ion shifts across the cell membrane, and refers to the cell's

PRELOAD AND AFTERLOAD

Preload refers to the blood's passive stretching of the ventricular muscle fibers at the end of diastole. According to Starling's law, the more the cardiac muscles are stretched in diastole, the more forcefully they contract in systole.

Afterload refers to the pressure that the ventricles need to generate to overcome higher pressure in the aorta so that blood can be ejected into the systemic circulation. This systemic vascular resistance corresponds to the systemic systolic pressure.

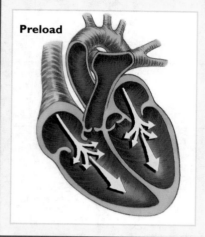

Preload

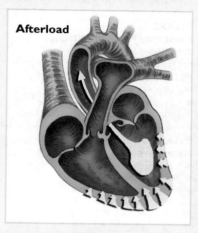

Afterload

---

ability to respond to an electrical stimulus. Conductivity is the ability of a cell to transmit an electrical impulse from one cell to another. Contractility refers to the cell's ability to contract after receiving a stimulus, by shortening and lengthening its muscle fibers.

The first three characteristics are electrical properties of the cells, while contractility represents a mechanical response to the electrical activity. Of the four characteristics, automaticity has the strongest effect on the genesis of cardiac rhythms.

DEPOLARIZATION AND REPOLARIZATION

As impulses are transmitted, cardiac cells undergo cycles of depolarization and repolarization. (See *Depolarization-*

repolarization cycle, page 14.) Cardiac cells at rest are considered to be polarized, meaning that no electrical activity takes place. Cell membranes separate concentrations of ions, such as sodium and potassium, and create a more negative charge inside the cell. This is called the resting potential. After a stimulus occurs, ions cross the cell membrane and trigger an action potential, or cell depolarization. When a cell is fully depolarized, it tries to return to its resting state in a process called repolarization. Electrical charges in the cell reverse and return to normal.

Phases of depolarization–repolarization

A depolarization-repolarization cycle consists of five phases numbered 0

DEPOLARIZATION-REPOLARIZATION CYCLE

The depolarization-repolarization cycle consists of the following phases:

PHASE 0:
RAPID DEPOLARIZATION
- Sodium (Na+) moves rapidly into cell.
- Calcium (Ca++) moves slowly into cell.

PHASE 1:
EARLY REPOLARIZATION
- Sodium channels close.

PHASE 2:
PLATEAU PHASE
- Calcium continues to flow in.
- Potassium (K+) continues to flow out.

PHASE 3:
RAPID REPOLARIZATION
- Calcium channels close.
- Potassium flows out rapidly.
- Active transport via the sodium-potassium pump begins restoring potassium to the inside of the cell and sodium to the outside of the cell.

PHASE 4:
RESTING PHASE
- Cell membrane is impermeable to sodium.
- Potassium moves out of the cell.

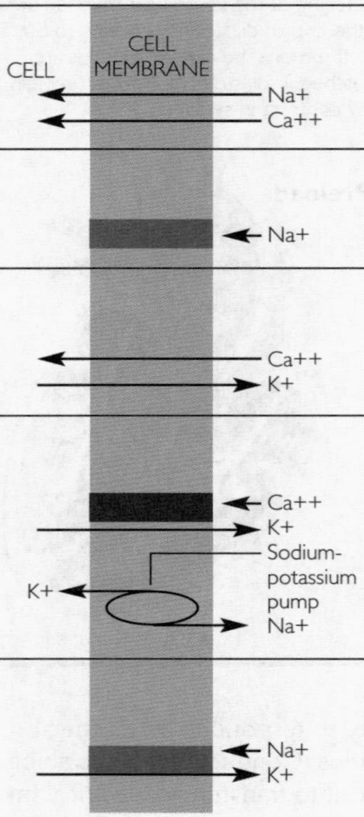

CELL   CELL MEMBRANE

Na+
Ca++

Na+

Ca++
K+

Ca++
K+
Sodium-potassium pump
K+
Na+

Na+
K+

---

through 4. A curve that shows voltage changes during the five phases represents the action potential. (See *Action potential curves.*)

During phase 0 (rapid depolarization), the cell receives a stimulus, usually from a neighboring cell. The cell becomes more permeable to sodium, the inside of the cell becomes less negative, the cell is depolarized, and myocardial contraction occurs. In phase 1 (early repolarization), sodium stops flowing into the cell, and the transmembrane potential falls slightly. Phase 2 (the plateau phase) is a pro-longed period of slow repolarization, when little change occurs in the cell's transmembrane potential.

During phases 1 and 2 and at the beginning of phase 3, the cardiac cell is in its absolute refractory period. During that period, no stimulus—no matter how strong—can excite the cell.

Phase 3 (rapid repolarization) occurs as the cell returns to its original state. During the last half of this phase, when the cell is in its relatively refractory period, a very strong stimulus can depolarize it.

ACTION POTENTIAL CURVES

An action potential curve shows the changes in a cell's electrical charge during the five phases of the depolarization-repolarization cycle. These graphs show electrical changes for nonpacemaker and pacemaker cells.

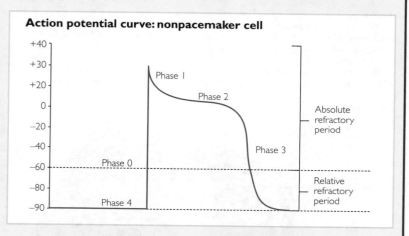

Action potential curve: nonpacemaker cell

As the graph shows, the action potential curve for pacemaker cells, such as those in the sinoatrial node, differs from that of other myocardial cells. Pacemaker cells have a resting membrane potential of −60 mV (instead of −90 mV), and they begin to depolarize spontaneously. Called *diastolic depolarization*, this effect is caused primarily by calcium and sodium leakage into the cell.

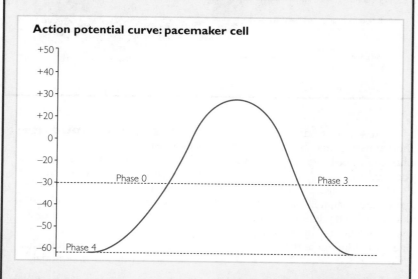

Action potential curve: pacemaker cell

CARDIAC CONDUCTION SYSTEM

The conduction system of the heart, as shown below, begins with the heart's dominant pacemaker, the sinoatrial (SA) node. The intrinsic rate of the SA node is 60 to 100 beats/minute. When an impulse leaves the SA node, it travels through the atria along Bachmann's bundle and the internodal pathways, on its way to the atrioventricular (AV) node and ventricles.

After the impulse passes through the AV node, it travels to the ventricles—first down the bundle of His, then along the bundle branches, and finally down the Purkinje fibers. Pacemaker cells in the junctional tissue and Purkinje fibers of the ventricles normally remain dormant because they receive impulses from the SA node. They initiate an impulse only when they don't receive one from the SA node. The intrinsic rate of the AV junction is 40 to 60 beats/minute; the intrinsic rate of the ventricles is 20 to 40 beats/minute.

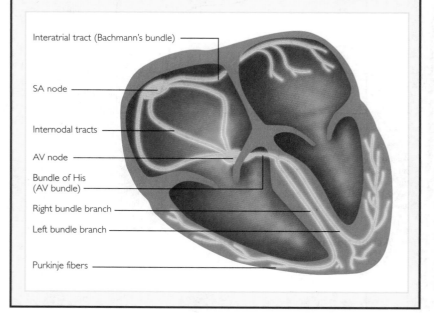

Interatrial tract (Bachmann's bundle)

SA node

Internodal tracts

AV node

Bundle of His
(AV bundle)

Right bundle branch

Left bundle branch

Purkinje fibers

Phase 4 is the resting phase of the action potential. By the end of phase 4, the cell is ready for another stimulus.

The electrical activity of the heart is represented on an ECG. Keep in mind that the ECG represents electrical activity only, not the mechanical activity or actual pumping of the heart.

ELECTRICAL CONDUCTION SYSTEM

After depolarization and repolarization occur, the resulting electric impulse travels through the heart along a pathway called the electrical conduction system. (See *Cardiac conduction system*.)

Impulses travel out from the SA node and through the internodal tracts and Bachmann's bundle to the AV node. From there, impulses travel through the bundle of His, the bundle branches, and finally to the Purkinje fibers.

SA node

The SA node, located in the right atrium where the superior vena cava joins the atrial tissue mass, is the heart's main pacemaker. Under resting conditions, the SA node generates impulses at a rate of 60 to 100 beats/minute. When initiated, the impulses follow a specific path through the heart. Electrical impulses usually don't travel backward because the cells can't respond to a stimulus immediately after depolarizing.

From the SA node, the impulse travels through the right and left atria. In the right atrium, the impulse is believed to be transmitted along three internodal tracts, sometimes referred to as the interatrial tracts. These include:
- anterior
- middle (Wenckebach's)
- posterior (Thorel's) internodal tracts.

The impulse travels through the left atrium via Bachmann's bundle, which are tracts of tissue that extend from the SA node to the left atrium. Impulse transmission through the right and left atria occurs so rapidly that the atria contract almost simultaneously.

AV node

The AV node is located in the inferior right atrium near the ostium of the coronary sinus. Although the AV node doesn't have pacemaker cells, the tissue surrounding it, called *junctional tissue,* contains pacemaker cells that can

fire at a rate of 40 to 60 beats/minute. As the AV node conducts the atrial impulse to the ventricles, it causes a 0.04-second delay. This delay allows the ventricles to complete their filling phase as the atria contract. It also allows the cardiac muscle to stretch to its fullest for peak cardiac output.

Bundle of His and bundle branches

Rapid conduction then resumes through the bundle of His, which separates into the right and left bundle branches. The branches extend down both sides of the interventricular septum:
- the right bundle branch extends down the right side of the interventricular septum and through the right ventricle
- the left bundle branch extends down the left side of the interventricular septum and through the left ventricle.

As a pacemaker site, the bundle of His has a firing rate of 40 to 60 beats/minute; it usually fires when the SA node fails to generate an impulse at a normal rate or when the impulse fails to reach the AV junction.

The left bundle branch then splits into two branches, or fasciculations:
- the left anterior fasciculus extends through the anterior portion of the left ventricle
- the left posterior fasciculus extends through the lateral and posterior portions of the left ventricle.

Impulses travel much faster down the left bundle branch, which feeds the larger, thicker-walled left ventricle, than the right bundle branch, which feeds the smaller, thinner-walled right ventricle. The difference in the conduction speed allows both

How reentry develops

Normally, conduction occurs along a single pathway, so reentry can't occur. In some people though, conduction occurs along two pathways—one fast and one slow. The speed and frequency of impulse conduction varies along those paths.

One pathway has a perfect surface for speed; the other pathway meanders through an obstacle course. Once an impulse starts off, it stays together until the pathways diverge.

Unidirectional conduction

When the pathways diverge, the impulses split up, as shown here. Half of the impulses take the fast pathway, and half struggle through obstacles on the slow pathway. The fast-pathway impulses reach the end point well ahead of the slow-pathway impulses, which causes the slow-pathway impulses to stop moving and disperse.

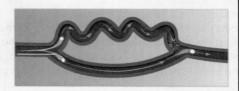

Premature impulse

If an ectopic impulse reaches the pathways prematurely, the fast pathway isn't ready; it's still refractory from the previous conduction. In such cases, as shown here, the impulse takes the slow pathway, which can accept impulses more quickly.

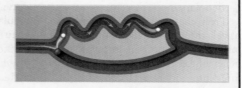

Reentry

When the impulses reach the bottom of the slow pathway, as shown here, one impulse splits off and heads to the end point. The others head back up the fast pathway. The impulse then continues around the circuit—down the slow pathway and up the fast pathway—repeatedly, sending one impulse each time to the end point and one back up to the starting point. That continuous looping of an impulse through the two pathways, known as *reentry*, can result in tachyarrhythmias.

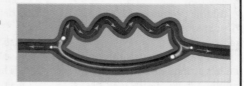

ventricles to contract at the same time. The entire network of specialized nervous tissue that extends through the ventricles is called the His-Purkinje system.

Purkinje system

Purkinje fibers—part of a diffuse muscle fiber network located under the endocardium—transmit impulses quicker than any other part of the conduction system. This pacemaker site usually doesn't fire unless the SA and AV nodes fail to generate an impulse or when the normal impulse is blocked in both bundle branches. The automatic firing rate of the Purkinje fibers ranges from 15 to 40 beats/minute.

In children younger than age 3, the AV node may discharge impulses 50 to 80 times/minute; the Purkinje fibers may discharge 40 to 50 times/minute.

Abnormal impulse conduction

Causes of abnormal impulse conduction include altered automaticity, retrograde conduction of impulses, reentry, and ectopy.

Altered automaticity

Automaticity, a special characteristic of pacemaker cells, allows them to trigger electrical impulses spontaneously. If a cell's automaticity increases or decreases, it can cause an arrhythmia (abnormality in the cardiac rhythm). Tachycardia and premature beats are commonly caused by an increase in the automaticity of pacemaker cells below the SA node. Likewise, a decrease in automaticity of cells in the SA node can lead to bradycardia or escape rhythms generated by lower pacemaker sites.

Retrograde conduction

Impulses that begin below the AV node can be transmitted back toward the atria. This backward (retrograde) conduction usually takes longer than normal conduction, and can cause the atria and ventricles to lose synchrony.

Reentry

Reentry occurs when cardiac tissue is activated two or more times by the same impulse. (See *How reentry develops.*) This may happen when conduction speed slows or when the refractory periods for neighboring cells occur at different times. Impulses are delayed long enough that cells have time to repolarize. In those cases, the active impulse reenters the same area and produces another impulse.

Ectopy

Pacemaker cells, when injured, may partially (rather than fully) depolarize. Partial depolarization can lead to spontaneous or secondary depolarization, or repetitive ectopic firings, called *triggered activity.* The resultant depolarization is called afterdepolarization. Early afterdepolarization occurs before the cell is fully repolarized and can be caused by hypokalemia, drug toxicity, or slow pacing rates. If it occurs after the cell has been fully repolarized, it's called *delayed afterdepolarization;* this may be caused by digoxin toxicity, hypercalcemia, or increased catecholamine release. This may result in atrial or ventricular tachycardias.

2
UNDERSTANDING ECGS

One of the most valuable diagnostic tools available, an electrocardiogram (ECG) records the heart's electrical activity as waveforms. By interpreting these waveforms accurately, you can identify rhythm disturbances, conduction abnormalities, and electrolyte imbalances. An ECG helps to diagnose and monitor conditions such as acute coronary syndromes and pericarditis.

To interpret an ECG correctly, you must first recognize its key components and analyze them separately before combining them to reach a conclusion about the heart's electrical activity. This chapter explains that analytic process, beginning with some fundamental information about electrocardiography.

The heart's electrical activity produces currents that radiate through the surrounding tissue to the skin. When electrodes are attached to the skin, they sense those electrical currents and transmit them to the electrocardiograph. This electrical activity is transformed into waveforms that represent the heart's depolarization-repolarization cycle.

Myocardial depolarization occurs when a wave of stimulation passes through the heart and causes the heart muscle to contract. Repolarization is the relaxation phase. An ECG shows the precise sequence of electrical events that occur in the cardiac cells throughout that process, and identifies rhythm disturbances and conduction abnormalities.

Leads and planes

Because the electrical currents from the heart radiate to the skin in many directions, electrodes are placed at different locations to obtain a total picture of the heart's electrical activity. The ECG can then record information from different perspectives, which are called *leads* and *planes*.

LEADS
A lead provides a view of the heart's electrical activity between two points, or poles. Each lead consists of one positive and one negative pole. Between the two poles lies an imaginary line representing the lead's axis, a term that refers to the direction of the current moving through the heart. Because each lead measures the heart's electrical potential from

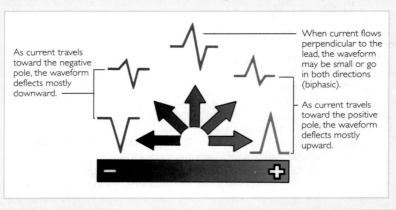
different directions, each generates its own characteristic tracing. (See *Current direction and waveform deflection*.)

The direction in which the electric current flows determines how the waveforms appear on the ECG tracing. When the current flows along the axis toward the positive pole of the electrode, the waveform deflects upward and is called a *positive deflection*. When the current flows away from the positive pole, the waveform deflects downward, below the baseline, and is called a *negative deflection*. When the current flows perpendicular to the axis, the wave may go in both directions or may be unusually small. When electrical activity is absent or too small to measure, the waveform is a straight line, also called an *isoelectric deflection*.

PLANES

A plane is a cross-section of the heart, which provides a different view of the heart's electrical activity. In the frontal plane—a vertical cut through the middle of the heart from top to bottom—electrical activity is viewed from right and left. The six limb leads are viewed from the frontal plane.

In the horizontal plane—a transverse cut through the middle of the heart dividing it into upper and lower portions—electrical activity can be seen moving toward the front and back. The six precordial leads are viewed from the horizontal plane.

Types of ECG recordings

The two main types of ECG recordings are the 12-lead ECG and the rhythm strip. Both types give valuable information about the heart's electrical activity.

12-LEAD ECG

A 12-lead ECG records information from 12 different views of the heart and provides a complete picture of electrical activity. These 12 views are obtained by placing electrodes on the patient's limbs and chest. The limb leads and the chest (*precordial*) leads reflect information from the different planes of the heart.

Different leads provide different information. The six limb leads—I, II, III, augmented vector right (aV_R), augmented vector left (aV_L), and augmented vector foot (aV_F)—provide information about the heart's frontal plane. Leads I, II, and III require a negative and positive electrode for monitoring, which makes these leads bipolar. The augmented leads—aV_R, aV_L, and aV_F—are unipolar, meaning they need only a positive electrode.

The six precordial (V) leads—V_1, V_2, V_3, V_4, V_5, and V_6—provide information about the heart's horizontal plane. Like the augmented leads, the precordial leads are unipolar, requiring only a positive electrode. The negative pole of these leads, which is in the center of the heart, is calculated with the ECG.

RHYTHM STRIP

A rhythm strip provides information about the heart's electric activity from one or more leads simultaneously and can be used to monitor cardiac status. Chest electrodes pick up the heart's electrical activity for display on a monitor. The monitor also displays heart rate and other measurements and prints out cardiac rhythm strips. Commonly monitored leads include leads II, V_1, and V_6.

Electrode placement

Electrode placement is different for each lead, and different leads provide different views of the heart. A lead may be chosen to highlight a particular part of the ECG complex or the electrical events of a specific area of the heart.

Although leads II, V_1, and V_6 are among the most commonly used leads for continuous monitoring, lead selection varies according to the patient's clinical status.

STANDARD LIMB LEADS

All standard limb leads or bipolar limb leads have a third electrode, known as the *ground,* which is placed on the chest to prevent electrical interference from appearing on the ECG recording. The axes of the three bipolar limb leads—I, II, and III—form a triangle around the heart and provide a frontal plane view of the heart. (See *Einthoven's triangle.*)

Lead I

Lead I provides a view of the heart that shows current moving from right to left. Because current flows from negative to positive, the positive electrode for this lead is placed on the left arm or on the left side of the chest; the negative electrode is placed on the right arm. Lead I produces a positive deflection on ECG tracings and is helpful in monitoring atrial rhythms.

Lead II

Lead II produces a positive deflection. The positive electrode is placed on the patient's left leg and the negative electrode on the right arm. For continuous monitoring, the electrodes are placed on the patient's torso for convenience,

EINTHOVEN'S TRIANGLE

The axes of the three bipolar limb leads (I, II, and III) form a triangle, known as *Einthoven's triangle*. Because the electrodes for these leads are about equidistant from the heart, the triangle is equilateral.

The axis of lead I extends from shoulder to shoulder; the right arm lead is the negative electrode, and the left arm lead is the positive electrode. The axis of lead II runs from the negative right arm lead electrode to the positive left leg lead electrode. The axis of lead III extends from the negative left arm lead electrode to the positive left leg lead electrode.

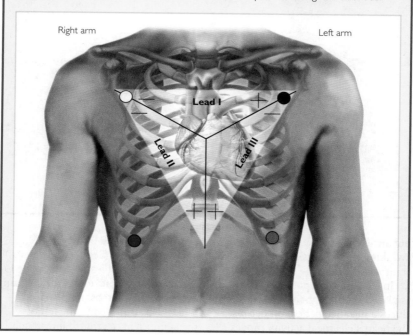

with the positive electrode below the lowest palpable rib at the left midclavicular line and the negative electrode below the right clavicle. The current travels down and to the left in this lead. Lead II tends to produce a positive, high-voltage deflection, resulting in tall P, R, and T waves. This lead is commonly used for routine monitoring and can help detect sinus node and atrial arrhythmias and monitor the inferior wall of the left ventricle.

Lead III
Lead III usually produces a positive deflection. The positive electrode is placed on the left leg and the negative electrode on the left arm. Along with lead II, this lead is useful for detecting changes associated with an inferior wall of the left ventricle.

AUGMENTED UNIPOLAR LEADS
Leads aV_R, aV_L, and aV_F are called *augmented leads* because the ECG

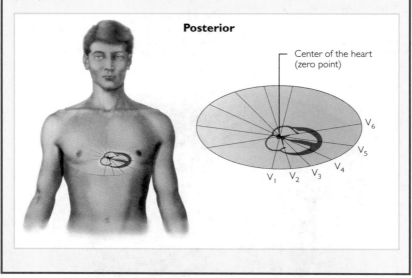

PRECORDIAL VIEWS

These illustrations show the different views of the heart obtained from each precordial (chest) lead.

Posterior

Center of the heart (zero point)

V_6
V_5
V_4
V_3
V_2
V_1

enhances the small waveforms that would normally appear from these unipolar leads.

In lead aV_R, the positive electrode is placed on the right arm and produces a negative deflection because the heart's electrical activity moves away from the lead. In lead aV_L, the positive electrode is on the left arm and usually produces a positive deflection on the ECG. In lead aV_F, the positive electrode is on the left leg (despite the name aV_F) and produces a positive deflection. These three limb leads also provide a view of the heart's frontal plane.

PRECORDIAL UNIPOLAR LEADS

The six unipolar *precordial leads* are placed in sequence across the chest

and provide a view of the heart's horizontal plane. (See *Precordial views*.)

The precordial lead V_1 electrode is placed on the right side of the sternum at the fourth intercostal rib space.

Lead V_2 is placed to the left of the sternum at the fourth intercostal space.

Lead V_3 goes between V_2 and V_4 at the fifth intercostal space. Leads V_1, V_2, and V_3 are biphasic, with positive and negative deflections.

Lead V_4 is placed at the fifth intercostal space at the midclavicular line and produces a positive deflection.

Lead V_5 is placed between leads V_4 and V_6 anterior to the axillary line, and produces a positive deflection on the ECG.

Lead V_6, the last of the precordial leads, is placed level with lead V_4 at the midaxillary line. Lead V_6 produces a positive deflection on the ECG.

These precordial leads are useful for monitoring ventricular arrhythmias, ST-segment changes, and bundle-branch blocks.

MODIFIED CHEST LEADS

If only a three-lead system is available, two other leads called MCL_1 and MCL_6 (modified chest leads) may be monitored. These two leads are similar to the unipolar leads V_1 and V_6 of the 12-lead ECG. However, MCL_1 and MCL_6 are bipolar leads. The modification of the chest lead occurs because a negative electrode is placed on the left side of the chest, rather than having the center of the heart function as the negative lead. MCL_1 is created by placing the negative electrode on the left upper chest, the positive electrode on the right side of the heart, and the ground electrode usually on the right upper chest. The MCL_1 lead most closely approximates the ECG pattern produced by the chest lead V_1.

When the positive electrode is on the right side of the heart and the electrical current travels toward the left ventricle, the waveform has a negative deflection. As a result, abnormal (ectopic) beats deflect in a positive direction.

Best lead *Choose MCL_1 to assess QRS-complex arrhythmias as a bipolar substitute for V_1. You can use this lead to monitor premature ventricular beats and to distinguish different types of tachycardia, such as ventricular and supraventricular tachycardia. MCL_1 can also be used to assess bundle-branch defects and P-wave changes and to confirm pacemaker wire placement.*

MCL_6 is an alternative to MCL_1 and most closely approximates the ECG pattern produced by the chest lead V_6. Like MCL_1, it monitors ventricular conduction changes. The positive lead in MCL_6 is placed at the midaxillary line of the left fifth intercostal space, the negative electrode below the left shoulder, and the ground below the right shoulder.

Examining the ECG grid

Waveforms produced by the heart's electrical current are recorded by a stylus on graphed ECG paper, which consists of horizontal and vertical lines that form a grid. A piece of ECG paper is called an *ECG strip* or *tracing*. (See *ECG grid,* page 26.)

The horizontal axis of the ECG strip represents time. Each small block equals 0.04 second, and five small blocks form a large block, which equals 0.20 second. This time increment is determined by multiplying 0.04 second (for one small block) by five, the number of small blocks that make up a large block. Five large blocks equal 1 second (5×0.20). When measuring or calculating a patient's heart rate, a 6-second strip consisting of 30 large blocks is usually used.

The ECG strip's vertical axis measures amplitude in millimeters (mm) or electrical voltage in millivolts (mV). Each small block represents 1 mm or 0.1 mV; each large block, 5 mm or 0.5 mV. To determine the amplitude of a wave, segment, or interval, count the number of small blocks from the baseline to the highest or lowest point of the wave, segment, or interval.

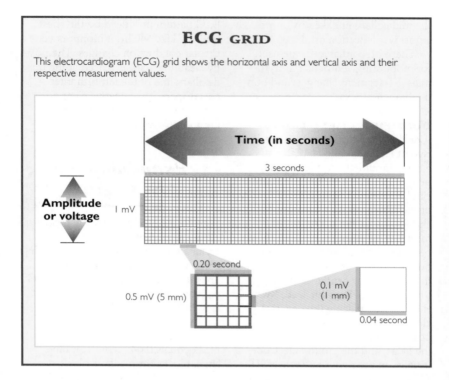

ECG GRID

This electrocardiogram (ECG) grid shows the horizontal axis and vertical axis and their respective measurement values.

Time (in seconds)

3 seconds

Amplitude or voltage

1 mV

0.20 second

0.5 mV (5 mm)

0.1 mV (1 mm)

0.04 second

ECG waveform components

An ECG complex characterizes the heart's electrical activity (the depolarization-repolarization cycle) that occurs in one cardiac cycle. The ECG tracing consists of three basic waveforms: the P wave, the QRS complex, and the T wave. These units of electrical activity can be further broken down into these segments and intervals: the PR interval, the ST segment, and the QT interval.

In addition, a U wave sometimes may be present. The J point marks the end of the QRS complex and the beginning of the ST segment. (See *ECG waveform components*.)

The upward and downward movement of the ECG's stylus, which forms the various waves, reflects the directional flow of the heart's electrical impulse. When the electrodes are placed correctly, an upward deflection is positive and a downward deflection is negative. Between each cardiac cycle, when the heart's electrical activity is absent, the stylus on the ECG recorder returns to the baseline or isoelectric line and records a straight line.

P WAVE

The P wave is the first component of a normal ECG waveform. It represents atrial depolarization, or conduction of an electrical impulse through the atria. When evaluating a P wave, look closely at its characteristics,

ECG WAVEFORM COMPONENTS

This illustration shows the components of a normal electrocardiogram (ECG) waveform.

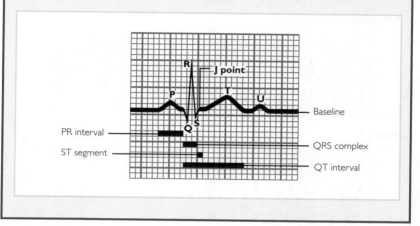

especially its location, configuration, and deflection. A normal P wave has the following characteristics.

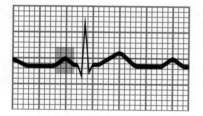

- *Location:* precedes the QRS complex
- *Amplitude:* 2 to 3 mm high
- *Duration:* 0.06 to 0.12 second
- *Configuration:* usually rounded and upright
- *Deflection:* positive or upright in leads I, II, aVF, and V_2 to V_6; usually positive but may vary in leads III and aVL; negative or inverted in lead aVR; biphasic or variable in lead V_1

If the deflection and configuration of a P wave are normal—for example, if the P wave is upright in lead II and is rounded and smooth—and if the P

wave precedes each QRS complex, you can assume that this electrical impulse originated in the sinoatrial (SA) node. The atria start to contract partway through the P wave, but you won't see this on the ECG. Remember, the ECG records only electrical activity, not mechanical activity or contraction.

Peaked, notched, or enlarged P waves may represent atrial hypertrophy or enlargement associated with chronic obstructive pulmonary disease, pulmonary emboli, valvular disease, or heart failure. Inverted P waves may signify retrograde or reverse conduction from the atrioventricular (AV) junction toward the atria. Whenever an upright sinus P wave becomes inverted, consider retrograde conduction and reverse conduction as possible conditions. (See *P-wave variations*, page 28.)

P-WAVE VARIATIONS

A P wave may be configured on lead II in the following ways:

Notched

Peaked

Inverted

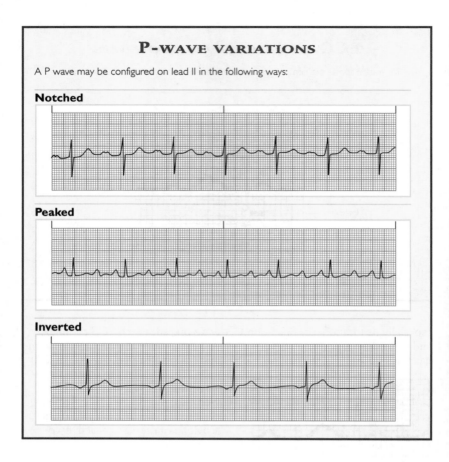

P-wave variations indicate that the impulse may be coming from different sites, such as from a wandering pacemaker rhythm, irritable atrial tissue, or damage near the SA node. Absence of P waves may signify impulse initiation by tissue other than the SA node, such as with a junctional or atrial fibrillation rhythm. When a P wave doesn't precede the QRS complex, there may be a heart block.

PR INTERVAL
The PR interval tracks the atrial impulse from the atria through the AV node and bundle of His. When evaluating a PR interval, look particularly at its duration. Changes in the PR interval indicate an altered impulse formation or a conduction delay, as seen in AV block. A normal PR interval has the following characteristics (amplitude, configuration, and deflection aren't measured):

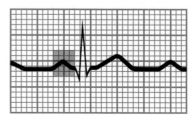

- *Location:* from the beginning of the P wave to the beginning of the QRS complex
- *Duration:* 0.12 to 0.20 second

Short PR intervals (shorter than 0.12 second) indicate that the impulse originated somewhere other than the SA node. This variation is associated with junctional arrhythmias and pre-excitation syndromes. Prolonged PR intervals (greater than 0.20 second) may represent a conduction delay through the atria or AV junction caused by digoxin toxicity, heart block, slowing related to ischemia, or conduction tissue disease.

QRS COMPLEX

The QRS complex follows the P wave and represents depolarization of the ventricles (*impulse conduction*). Immediately after the ventricles depolarize, as represented by the QRS complex, they contract. That contraction ejects blood from the ventricles and pumps it through the arteries, creating a pulse.

Whenever you're monitoring cardiac rhythm, remember that the waveform you see represents only the heart's electrical activity. It doesn't guarantee a mechanical contraction of the heart and a subsequent pulse. The contraction could be weak, as happens with premature ventricular contractions, or absent, as happens with pulseless electrical activity. So check the patient before you treat what the strip shows. Pay special attention to the duration and configuration when evaluating a QRS complex. A normal complex has the following characteristics:

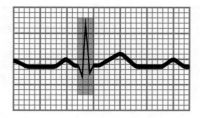

- *Location:* follows the PR interval
- *Amplitude:* 5 to 30 mm high, but differs for each lead used
- *Duration:* 0.06 to 0.10 second or half of the PR interval (duration is measured from the beginning of the Q wave to the end of the S wave, or from the beginning of the R wave if the Q wave is absent)
- *Configuration*: Consists of the Q wave (the first negative deflection, or deflection below the baseline, after the P wave), the R wave (the first positive deflection after the Q wave), and the S wave (the first negative deflection after the R wave); you may not always see all three waves and it may look different for each lead (see *QRS waveform variety,* page 30)
- *Deflection:* positive (with most of the complex above the baseline) in leads I, II, III, aV_L, aV_F, and V_4 to V_6, negative in leads aV_R and V_1 to V_2, and biphasic in lead V_3

Remember that the QRS complex represents intraventricular conduction time. That's why identifying and correctly interpreting it is so crucial. If no P wave appears with the QRS complex, then the impulse may have originated in the ventricles, indicating a ventricular arrhythmia.

Deep, wide Q waves may indicate that a myocardial infarction has occurred. In this case, the Q-wave am-

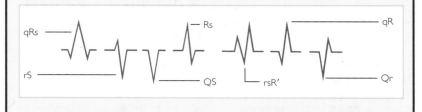
plitude (depth) is greater than or equal to 25% of the height of the succeeding R wave, or the duration of the Q wave is 0.04 second or more. A notched R wave may signify a bundle-branch block. A widened QRS complex (greater than 0.12 second) may signify a ventricular conduction delay. A missing QRS complex may indicate AV block or ventricular standstill.

ST SEGMENT

The ST segment represents the end of ventricular conduction or depolarization and the beginning of ventricular recovery or repolarization. The point that marks the end of the QRS complex and the beginning of the ST segment is known as the *J point.*

Pay special attention to the deflection of an ST segment. A normal ST segment has the following characteristics (amplitude, duration, and configuration aren't observed):

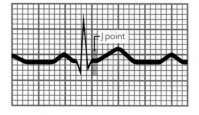

● *Location:* extends from the S wave to the beginning of the T wave
● *Deflection:* usually isoelectric or on the baseline (neither positive nor negative); may vary from -0.5 to +1 mm in some precordial leads

A change in the ST segment may indicate myocardial injury or ischemia. An ST segment may become either elevated or depressed. (See *Changes in the ST segment.*)

T WAVE

The peak of the T wave represents the relative refractory period of repolarization or ventricular recovery. When evaluating a T wave, look at the amplitude, configuration, and deflection.

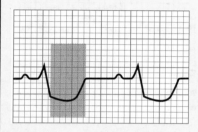 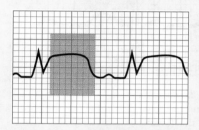
Normal T waves have the following characteristics (duration isn't measured).

- *Location:* follows the ST segment

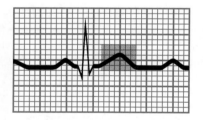

- *Amplitude:* 0.5 mm in leads I, II, and III and up to 10 mm in the precordial leads
- *Configuration:* typically rounded and smooth
- *Deflection:* usually positive or upright in leads I, II, and V_2 to V_6; inverted in lead aV_R; variable in leads III and V_1

The T wave's peak represents the relative refractory period of ventricular repolarization, a period during which cells are especially vulnerable to extra stimuli. Bumps in a T wave may indicate that a P wave is hidden in it. If a P wave is hidden, atrial depolarization has occurred, the impulse having originated at a site above the ventricles.

Tall, peaked, or "tented" T waves may indicate myocardial injury or electrolyte imbalances such as hyperkalemia. Inverted T waves in leads I, II, aV_L, aV_F, or V_2 through V_6 may represent myocardial ischemia. Heavily notched or pointed T waves in an adult may indicate pericarditis.

QT INTERVAL

The QT interval measures the time needed for ventricular depolarization and repolarization. The length of the QT interval varies according to heart rate. The faster the heart rate, the shorter the QT interval. When checking the QT interval, look closely at the duration.

A normal QT interval has the following characteristics (amplitude, configuration, and deflection aren't observed).

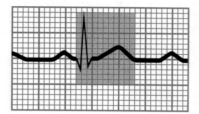

- *Location:* extends from the beginning of the QRS complex to the end of the T wave
- *Duration:* varies according to age, gender, and heart rate; usually lasts from 0.36 to 0.44 second; shouldn't be greater than half the distance between the two consecutive R waves (called the *R-R interval*) when the rhythm is regular

The QT interval measures the time needed for ventricular depolarization and repolarization. Prolonged QT intervals indicate that ventricular repolarization time is slowed, meaning that the relative refractory (vulnerable) period of the cardiac cycle is longer.

Prolonged QT syndrome is a congenital conduction-system defect present in certain families. This variation is also associated with certain medications, such as class I antiarrhythmics. Short QT intervals may result from digoxin toxicity or electrolyte imbalances such as hypercalcemia.

U WAVE

The U wave represents repolarization of the His-Purkinje system or ventricu-

lar conduction fibers. It isn't present on every rhythm strip. The configuration is the most important characteristic of the U wave.

When present, a normal U wave has the following characteristics (amplitude and duration aren't measured).

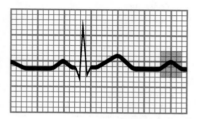

- *Location:* follows the T wave
- *Configuration:* typically upright and rounded
- *Deflection:* upright

The U wave may not appear on an ECG. A prominent U wave may be caused by hypercalcemia, hypokalemia, or digoxin toxicity.

Normal sinus rhythm

You must be able to recognize a normal cardiac rhythm before you can recognize an arrhythmia. The term *arrhythmia* literally means "an absence of rhythm," but the more accurate term, *dysrhythmia,* means "an abnormality in rhythm." However, these terms are typically used interchangeably.

Normal sinus rhythm (NSR) occurs when an impulse starts in the sinus node and progresses to the ventricles through a normal conduction pathway—from the sinus node to the atria and AV node, through the bundle of His to the bundle branches, and on to the Purkinje fibers. No premature or aberrant contractions are present. NSR

RECOGNIZING NORMAL SINUS RHYTHM

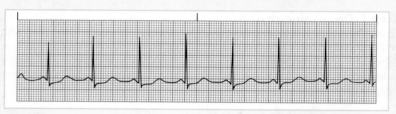

RHYTHM
- Atrial regular
- Ventricular regular

RATE
- 60 to 100 beats/minute (sinoatrial node's normal firing rate)

P WAVE
- Normal shape (round and smooth)
- Upright in lead II
- One for every QRS complex
- All similar in size and shape

PR INTERVAL
- Within normal limits (0.12 to 0.20 second)

QRS COMPLEX
- Within normal limits (0.06 to 0.10 second)

T WAVE
- Normal shape
- Upright and rounded in lead II

QT INTERVAL
- Within normal limits (0.36 to 0.44 second)

OTHER
- No ectopic or aberrant beats

---

is the standard against which all other rhythms are compared. (See *Recognizing normal sinus rhythm*.)

Practice the eight-step method, described below, to analyze an ECG strip with a normal cardiac rhythm (NSR). The ECG characteristics of NSR include:
- *Rhythm*—atrial and ventricular rhythms are regular
- *Rate*—atrial and ventricular rates are 60 to 100 beats/minute, the SA node's normal firing rate
- *P wave*—normal shape (round and smooth) and upright in lead II; all P waves similar in size and shape; one P wave for every QRS complex

- *PR interval*—within normal limits (0.12 to 0.20 second)
- *QRS complex*—within normal limits (0.06 to 0.10 second)
- *T wave*—normal shape; upright and rounded in lead II
- *QT interval*—within normal limits (0.36 to 0.44 second)
- *Other*—no ectopic or aberrant beats.

THE EIGHT-STEP METHOD
Analyzing a rhythm strip is a skill developed through practice. You can use several methods, as long as you're consistent. Rhythm strip analysis requires a sequential and systematic ap-

proach, such as the eight steps described below.

Step 1: Determine rhythm

To determine the heart's atrial and ventricular rhythms, use either the paper-and-pencil method or the caliper method. (See *Methods of measuring rhythm*.)

For atrial rhythm, measure the P-P intervals—that is, the intervals between consecutive P waves. These intervals should occur regularly, with only small variations associated with respirations. Then compare the P-P intervals in several cycles. Consistently similar P-P intervals indicate regular

---

METHODS OF MEASURING RHYTHM

You can use either of the following methods to determine atrial or ventricular rhythm.

PAPER-AND-PENCIL METHOD
◆ Place the electrocardiogram (ECG) strip on a flat surface.
◆ Position the straight edge of a piece of paper along the strip's baseline.
◆ Move the paper up slightly so the straight edge is near the peak of the R wave.
◆ With a pencil, mark the paper at the R waves of two consecutive QRS complexes, as shown below. This distance is the R-R interval.
◆ Move the paper across the strip lining up the two marks with succeeding R-R intervals. If the distance for each R-R interval is the same, the ventricular rhythm is regular. If the distance varies, the rhythm is irregular.
◆ Use the same method to measure the distance between P waves (the P-P interval) and determine whether the atrial rhythm is regular or irregular.

CALIPER METHOD
◆ With the ECG on a flat surface, place one point of the calipers on the peak of the first R wave of two consecutive QRS complexes.
◆ Adjust the caliper legs so the other point is on the peak of the next R wave, as shown below. This distance is the R-R interval.
◆ Pivot the first point of the calipers toward the third R wave, and note whether it falls on the peak of that wave.
◆ Check succeeding R-R intervals in the same way. If they're all the same, the ventricular rhythm is regular. If they vary, the rhythm is irregular.
◆ Using the same method, measure the P-P intervals to determine whether the atrial rhythm is regular or irregular.

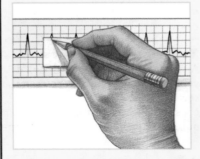

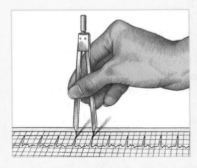

atrial rhythm; dissimilar P-P intervals indicate irregular atrial rhythm.

To determine the ventricular rhythm, measure the intervals between two consecutive R waves in the QRS complexes. If an R wave isn't present, use either the Q wave or the S wave of consecutive QRS complexes. The R-R intervals should occur regularly. Then compare R-R intervals in several cycles. As with atrial rhythms, consistently similar R-R intervals mean a regular ventricular rhythm; dissimilar R-R intervals point to an irregular ventricular rhythm.

After completing your measurements, ask yourself:
● Is the rhythm regular or irregular? Consider a rhythm with only slight variations, up to 0.04 second, to be regular.
● If the rhythm is irregular, is it slightly irregular or markedly so? Does the irregularity occur in a pattern (a regularly irregular pattern)?

Step 2: Calculate rate
You can use one of three methods to determine atrial and ventricular heart rates from an ECG waveform. Although these methods can provide accurate information, you shouldn't rely solely on them when assessing your patient. Keep in mind that the ECG waveform represents electrical, not mechanical, activity. Therefore, although an ECG can show you that ventricular depolarization has occurred, it doesn't mean that ventricular contraction has occurred. To determine this, you must assess the patient's pulse. So remember, always check a pulse to correlate it with the heart rate on the ECG.
● *Times-10 method:* This first method is the simplest, quickest, and most

common way to calculate rate, especially if the rhythm is irregular. ECG paper is marked in increments of 3 seconds, or 15 large boxes. To calculate the atrial rate, obtain a 6-second strip, count the number of P waves on it, and multiply by 10. Ten 6-second strips equal 1 minute. Calculate ventricular rate the same way, using the R waves.
● *1,500 method:* If the heart rhythm is regular, use this method, so named because 1,500 small squares equal 1 minute. Count the number of small squares between identical points on two consecutive P waves, and then divide 1,500 by that number to get the atrial rate. To obtain the ventricular rate, use the same method with two consecutive R waves.
● *Sequence method:* This third method of estimating heart rate requires memorizing a sequence of numbers. For atrial rate, find a P wave that peaks on a heavy black line and assign the following numbers to the next six heavy black lines: 300, 150, 100, 75, 60, and 50. Then find the next P-wave peak and estimate the atrial rate, based on the number assigned to the nearest heavy black line. Estimate the ventricular rate the same way, using the R wave. (See *Calculating heart rate,* page 36.)

Step 3: Evaluate P wave
When examining a rhythm strip for P waves, ask yourself:
● Are P waves present?
● Do the P waves have a normal configuration?
● Do all the P waves have a similar size and shape?
● Is there one P wave for every QRS complex?

CALCULATING HEART RATE

This table can help make the sequencing method of determining heart rate more precise. After counting the number of boxes between the R waves, use this table to find the rate.

For example, if you count 20 small blocks, or 4 large blocks, the rate would be 75 beats/minute. To calculate the atrial rate, use the same method with P waves instead of R waves.

RAPID ESTIMATION

This rapid-rate calculation is also called the *countdown method.* Using the number of large boxes between R waves or P waves as a guide, you can rapidly estimate ventricular or atrial rates by memorizing the sequence "300, 150, 100, 75, 60, 50."

NUMBER OF SMALL BLOCKS	HEART RATE
5 (1 large block)	300
6	250
7	214
8	188
9	167
10 (2 large blocks)	150
11	136
12	125
13	115
14	107
15 (3 large blocks)	100
16	94
17	88
18	83
19	79
20 (4 large blocks)	75
21	71
22	68
23	65
24	63
25 (5 large blocks)	60
26	58
27	56
28	54
29	52
30 (6 large blocks)	50
31	48
32	47
33	45
34	44
35 (7 large blocks)	43
36	42
37	41
38	39
39	38
40 (8 large blocks)	37

Step 4: Determine PR-interval duration

To measure the PR interval, count the small squares between the start of the P wave and the start of the QRS complex; then multiply the number of squares by 0.04 second. After performing this calculation, ask yourself:
● Does the duration of the PR interval fall within normal limits, 0.12 to 0.20 second (or 3 to 5 small squares)?
● Is the PR interval constant?

Step 5: Determine QRS-complex duration

When determining QRS-complex duration, make sure you measure straight across from the end of the PR interval to the end of the S wave, not just to the peak. Remember, the QRS complex has no horizontal components. To calculate duration, count the number of small squares between the beginning and end of the QRS complex and multiply this number by 0.04 second. Then ask yourself:
● Does the duration of the QRS complex fall within normal limits, 0.06 to 0.10 second?
● Are all QRS complexes the same size and shape? (If not, measure each one and describe them individually.)
● Does a QRS complex appear after every P wave?

Step 6: Evaluate T wave

Examine the T waves on the ECG strip. Then ask yourself:
● Are T waves present?
● Do all of the T waves have a normal shape?
● Could a P wave be hidden in a T wave?
● Do all T waves have a normal amplitude?
● Do the T waves have the same deflection as the QRS complexes?

Step 7: Determine QT-interval duration

Count the number of small squares between the beginning of the QRS complex and the end of the T wave, where the T wave returns to the baseline. Multiply this number by 0.04 second. Ask yourself:
● Does the duration of the QT interval fall within normal limits, 0.36 to 0.44 second?

Step 8: Evaluate other components

Note the presence of ectopic beats or other abnormalities, such as aberrant conduction. Also, check the ST segment for abnormalities, and look for the presence of a U wave.

Now, interpret your findings by classifying the rhythm strip according to one or all of the following:
● *Origin of the rhythm:* for example, sinus node, atria, AV node, or ventricles
● *Rate:* normal (60 to 100 beats/minute), bradycardia (less than 60 beats/minute), or tachycardia (more than 100 beats/minute)
● *Rhythm interpretation:* normal or abnormal; for example, flutter, fibrillation, heart block, escape rhythm, or other arrhythmias.

3

ECG MONITORING

The type of electrocardiogram (ECG) monitoring system used (hardwire monitoring or telemetry) depends on what is available in the facility and is often guided by the patient's condition.

Hardwire monitoring

With hardwire monitoring, the electrodes on the patient's chest connect to leadwire cable hooked directly to the bedside cardiac monitor. Most hardwire monitors are mounted permanently on a shelf or wall near the patient's bed, but some monitors are mounted on an I.V. pole for portability and have defibrillating and transcutaneous pacing capability.

The cardiac monitor provides a continuous cardiac rhythm display and transmits the ECG tracing to a console at the nurses' station. Both the monitor and the console have alarms that sound when the heart rate falls below or exceeds the set limits or when arrhythmias occur. Both can also print rhythm strips. Hardwire monitors usually have the ability to track:
- blood pressure
- hemodynamic measurements

- pulse oximetry
- other parameters through various attachments to the patient.

Intensive care units and emergency departments generally use hardwire monitoring because it permits continuous observation of one or more patients from more than one area in the unit. However, this type of monitoring does have disadvantages, including limited mobility because the patient is connected to the monitor.

Telemetry monitoring

With telemetry monitoring, the electrodes on the patient's chest connect to a lead wire cable that connects to a small, battery-powered transmitter carried in a pocket or pouch that sends electric signals to a central station, where the signals are displayed on a monitor screen. This type of ECG monitoring allows the patient greater mobility.

Telemetry monitoring is especially useful for detecting arrhythmias that occur at rest or during sleep, exercise, or stressful situations. However, most systems can monitor only heart rate and rhythm.

Leadwire systems

A three- or five-leadwire-electrode system may be used for bedside cardiac monitoring. (See *Leadwire systems,* pages 40 and 41.) Both systems use a ground wire to prevent accidental electrical shock to the patient.

A three-electrode system has one positive electrode, one negative electrode, and a ground. The popular five-electrode system has, in addition to those three electrodes, a right leg electrode that becomes a permanent ground for all leads and an exploratory chest lead that allows monitoring of any six modified chest leads as well as the standard limb leads. This system uses standardized chest placement. Wires that attach to the electrodes are usually color-coded to help you place them correctly on the patient's chest. Most five-lead systems provide continuous monitoring of two or more leads simultaneously. (See *Dual-lead monitoring,* page 41.)

One newer application of bedside cardiac monitoring is a reduced lead continuous 12-lead ECG system (EASI system).

This system uses an advanced algorithm and only five electrodes uniquely placed on the torso to derive a 12-lead ECG. The system allows all 12 leads to be simultaneously displayed and recorded. (See *Understanding the EASI system,* page 42.)

APPLICATION OF ELECTRODES

Before attaching electrodes to your patient, make sure he knows you're *monitoring* his heart rate and rhythm, not controlling them. Tell him not to become upset if he hears an alarm during the procedure; it probably just means a leadwire has come loose.

Explain the electrode placement procedure to the patient, provide privacy, and wash your hands. Expose the patient's chest and select electrode sites for the chosen lead. Choose sites over soft tissues or close to bone. Don't choose sites over bony prominences, thick muscles, or skin folds; those areas can produce ECG artifact (waveforms not produced by the heart's electrical activity).

Skin preparation

Prepare the patient's skin by doing the following:

● Wash the chest with soap and water and dry it thoroughly.
● Clip dense hair with clippers or scissors to prevent interference with electric contact.
● If the patient has oily skin, clean each site with an alcohol pad and let it air dry. This ensures proper adhesion and prevents alcohol from becoming trapped beneath the electrode, which can irritate or break down the skin.
● Use a special rough patch on the back of the electrode, a dry washcloth, or a gauze pad to briskly rub each site until the skin reddens but be careful not to damage or break the skin. Brisk scrubbing helps to remove dead skin cells and improves electrical contact.

Application of electrode pads

To apply the electrodes, remove the backing and make sure each pre-gelled electrode is still moist. If an electrode has become dry, discard it and select another. A dry electrode decreases electrical contact and interferes with waveforms.

(Text continues on page 42.)

LEADWIRE SYSTEMS

This chart shows the correct electrode positions for some of the leads that you'll use most often—the five-leadwire, three-leadwire, and telemetry systems. The chart uses the abbreviations RA for the right arm, LA for the left arm, RL for the right leg, LL for the left leg, C for the chest, and G for the ground.

ELECTRODE POSITIONS
In the three- and five-leadwire systems, electrode positions for one lead may be identical to those for another lead. When that happens, change the lead selector switch to the setting that corresponds to the lead you want. In some cases, you'll need to reposition the electrodes.

TELEMETRY
In a telemetry monitoring system, you can create the same leads as the other systems with just two electrodes and a ground wire.

FIVE-LEADWIRE SYSTEM	THREE-LEADWIRE SYSTEM	TELEMETRY SYSTEM
Lead I		

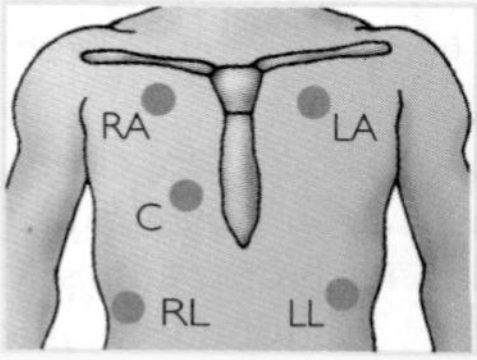

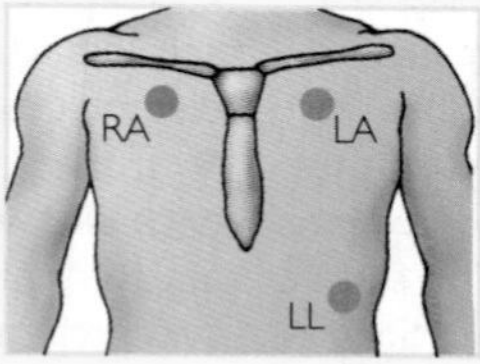

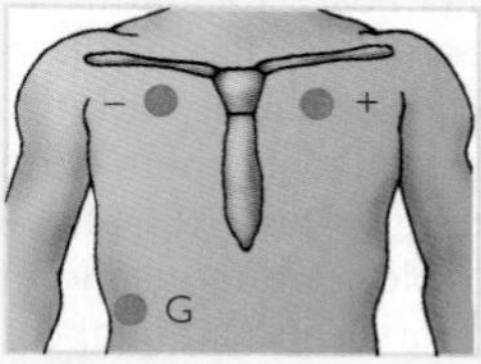

Lead II

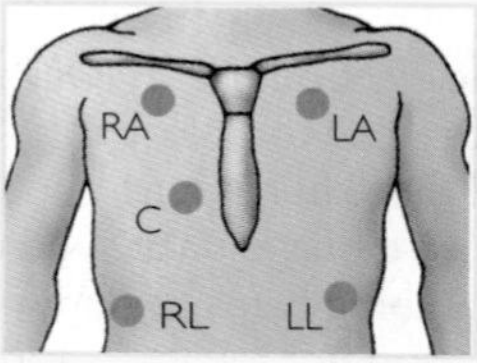

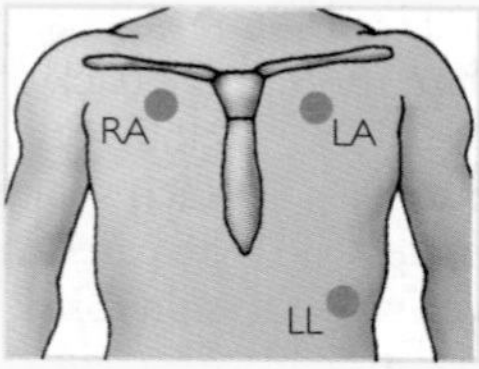

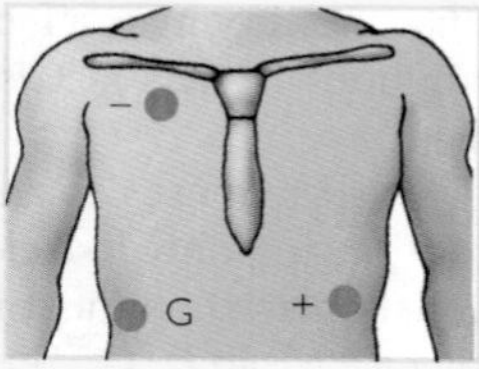

Lead III

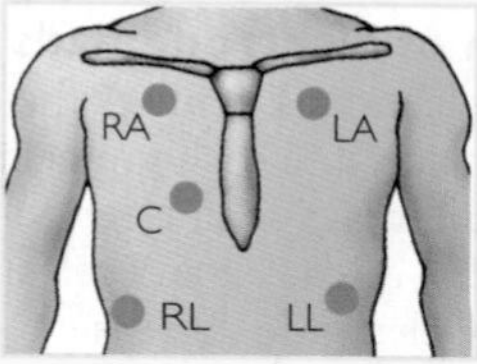

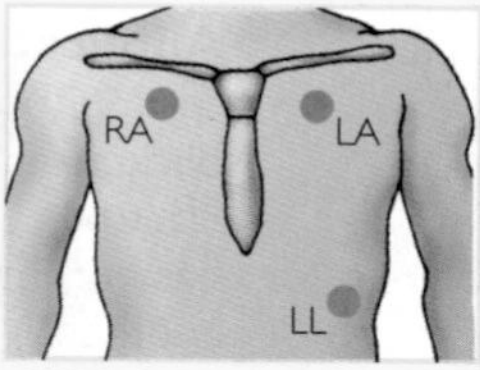

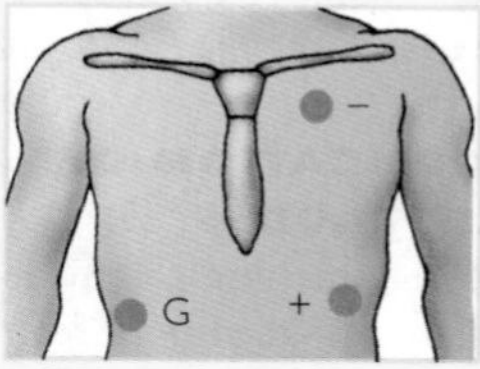

FIVE-LEADWIRE SYSTEM	THREE-LEADWIRE SYSTEM	TELEMETRY SYSTEM

Lead MCL$_1$

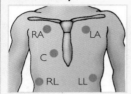 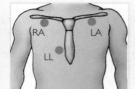 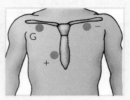

Lead MCL$_6$

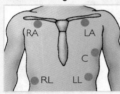 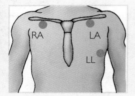 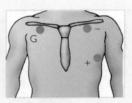

DUAL-LEAD MONITORING

Monitoring in two leads provides a more complete picture than does monitoring in one. Therefore, if it's available, dual-lead monitoring should be used to detect ectopy or aberrant rhythms.

Lead II

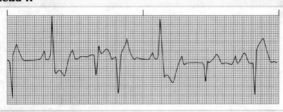

Lead V$_1$

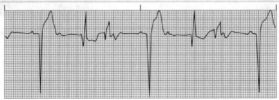

UNDERSTANDING THE EASI SYSTEM

The five-lead EASI (reduced lead continuous 12-lead electrocardiogram [ECG]) configuration gives a three-dimensional view of the electrical activity of the heart from the frontal, horizontal, and sagittal planes. This provides 12 leads of information. A mathematical calculation in the electronics of the monitoring system is applied to the information, creating a derived 12-lead ECG.

Placement of the electrodes for the EASI system includes:
- ◆ *E lead:* lower part of the sternum at the level of the fifth intercostal space
- ◆ *A lead:* left midaxillary line at the level of the fifth intercostal space
- ◆ *S lead:* upper part of the sternum
- ◆ *I lead:* right midaxillary line at the level of the fifth intercostal space
- ◆ *Ground:* anywhere on the torso

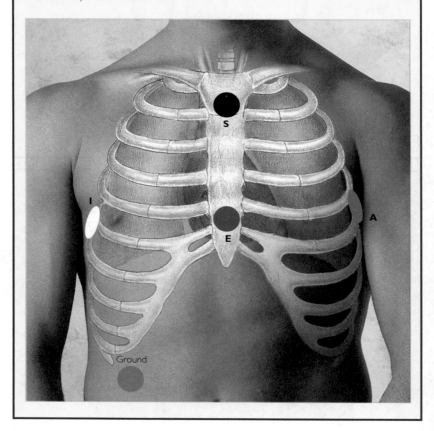

Apply one electrode to each prepared site using this method:

- Press one side of the electrode against the patient's skin, pull gently, and then press the opposite side of the electrode against the skin.

- Using two fingers, press the adhesive edge around the outside of the electrode to the patient's chest. This fixes the gel and stabilizes the electrode.
- Repeat this procedure for each electrode.
- Every 24 hours or according to your facility's policy and procedure, remove the electrodes, assess the patient's skin, and replace the old electrodes with new ones.

Attaching leadwires

You'll also need to attach leadwires and the cable connections to the monitor, and then attach leadwires to the electrodes. Leadwires may clip or (more often) snap on. If you're using the snap-on type, attach the electrode to the leadwire immediately before applying it to the patient's chest. When possible, do this step ahead of time to prevent patient discomfort and disturbances of the contact between the electrode and the skin. When you use a clip-on leadwire, apply it after the electrode has been secured to the patient's skin. That way, applying the clip won't interfere with the electrode's contact with the skin.

Observing cardiac rhythm

After the electrodes are properly positioned, the monitor is on, and the necessary cables are attached, observe the screen. You should see the patient's ECG waveform. Although some monitoring systems allow you to make adjustments by touching the screen, most require you to manipulate knobs and buttons. If the waveform appears too large or too small, change the size by adjusting the gain control. If the waveform appears too high or too low on the screen, adjust the position dial.

Verify that the monitor detects each heartbeat by comparing the patient's apical rate with the rate displayed on the monitor. Set the upper and lower limits of the heart rate according to your facility's policy and the patient's condition. Heart rate alarms are generally set 10 to 20 beats/minute higher or lower than the patient's heart rate.

Monitors with arrhythmia detection generate a rhythm strip automatically whenever the alarm goes off. Some cardiac monitoring systems use a portable paging system that alerts the nurse to potential arrhythmias. You can obtain other views of your patient's cardiac rhythm by selecting different leads. You can select leads with the lead selector button or switch.

To get a printout of the patient's cardiac rhythm, press the "record" control on the monitor. The ECG strip will be printed at the central console. Some systems print the rhythm from a recorder box on the monitor itself.

Most monitors allow you to add the patient's name, date, and time as a permanent record; if the monitor you're using doesn't have this capacity, label the rhythm strip with the patient's name, date, time, and rhythm interpretation. Add appropriate clinical information to the ECG strip, such as drug administered, presence of chest pain, or patient activity at the time of the recording. Be sure to place the rhythm strip in the appropriate section of the patient's medical record.

COMMON MONITOR PROBLEMS

These illustrations present the most commonly encountered monitor problems, including the way to identify them, their possible causes, and interventions.

WAVEFORM	POSSIBLE CAUSES	INTERVENTIONS
ARTIFACT (WAVEFORM INTERFERENCE) 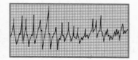	◆ Patient experiencing seizures, chills, or anxiety	◆ If the patient is having a seizure, notify the physician and intervene as ordered. ◆ Keep the patient warm and encourage him to relax.
	◆ Dirty or corroded connections	◆ Replace dirty or corroded wires.
	◆ Improper electrode application	◆ Check the electrodes, and reapply them if needed. Clean the patient's skin well, because skin oils and dead skin cells inhibit conduction.
	◆ Dry electrode gel	◆ Check the electrode gel. If the gel is dry, apply new electrodes.
	◆ Short circuit in lead-wires or cable	◆ Replace broken equipment.
	◆ Electrical interference from other equipment in the room	◆ Make sure all electrical equipment is attached to a common ground. Check all three-pronged plugs to ensure that no prong is loose. Notify biomedical department.
	◆ Static electricity interference from inadequate room humidity	◆ Keep room humidity at 40%, if possible.
FALSE HIGH-RATE ALARM 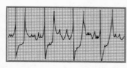	◆ Gain setting too high, particularly with MCL_1 setting	◆ Assess the patient for signs and symptoms of hyperkalemia. ◆ Reset gain.
	◆ HIGH alarm set too low or LOW alarm set too high	◆ Set alarm limits according to the patient's heart rate.
WEAK SIGNALS 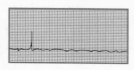	◆ Improper electrode application	◆ Reapply the electrodes.
	◆ QRS complex too small to register	◆ Reset gain so that the height of the complex is greater than 1 mV. ◆ Try monitoring the patient on another lead.
	◆ Wire or cable failure	◆ Replace any faulty wires or cables.

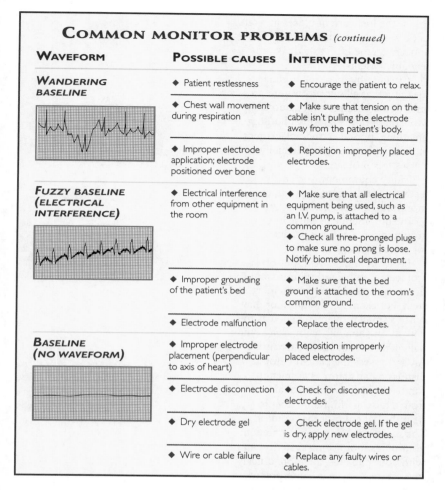

COMMON MONITOR PROBLEMS *(continued)*

WAVEFORM	POSSIBLE CAUSES	INTERVENTIONS
WANDERING BASELINE	◆ Patient restlessness	◆ Encourage the patient to relax.
	◆ Chest wall movement during respiration	◆ Make sure that tension on the cable isn't pulling the electrode away from the patient's body.
	◆ Improper electrode application; electrode positioned over bone	◆ Reposition improperly placed electrodes.
FUZZY BASELINE (ELECTRICAL INTERFERENCE)	◆ Electrical interference from other equipment in the room	◆ Make sure that all electrical equipment being used, such as an I.V. pump, is attached to a common ground. ◆ Check all three-pronged plugs to make sure no prong is loose. Notify biomedical department.
	◆ Improper grounding of the patient's bed	◆ Make sure that the bed ground is attached to the room's common ground.
	◆ Electrode malfunction	◆ Replace the electrodes.
BASELINE (NO WAVEFORM)	◆ Improper electrode placement (perpendicular to axis of heart)	◆ Reposition improperly placed electrodes.
	◆ Electrode disconnection	◆ Check for disconnected electrodes.
	◆ Dry electrode gel	◆ Check electrode gel. If the gel is dry, apply new electrodes.
	◆ Wire or cable failure	◆ Replace any faulty wires or cables.

Troubleshooting monitor problems

For optimal cardiac monitoring, you need to recognize problems that can interfere with obtaining a reliable ECG recording. (See *Common monitor problems*.) Causes of interference include patient movement and poorly placed or poorly functioning equipment.

An artifact, also called *waveform interference,* may occur with excessive movement (somatic tremor). It causes the baseline of the ECG to appear wavy, bumpy, or tremulous. Dry electrodes also may cause this problem because of poor contact.

Electrical interference, also called *AC interference* or *60-cycle interference,* is caused by electrical power leakage. It also may result from interference from other equipment in the room, or from improperly grounded equipment. As a result, the lost current pulses at a rate of 60 cycles/second. This interference appears on the ECG as a thick, unreadable baseline.

A wandering baseline undulates, meaning that all waveforms are present but the baseline isn't stationary. Movement of the chest wall during breathing, poor electrode placement, or poor electrode contact usually causes this problem.

Faulty equipment, such as broken leadwires and cables, also can cause monitoring problems. Excessively worn equipment can cause improper grounding, putting the patient at risk for accidental shock.

Be aware that some types of artifacts resemble arrhythmias and the monitor will interpret them as such. For example, the monitor may sense a small movement, such as the patient brushing his teeth, as a potentially lethal ventricular tachycardia. Always assess the patient before dismissing an alarm as artifact; it can be difficult to tell a real alarm from a false alarm. Remember to treat the patient, not the monitor. The more familiar you become with your unit's monitoring system—and with your patient—the more quickly you can recognize and interpret monitor problems and act appropriately.

PART 2

Intrepreting rhythm strips

4

SINOATRIAL NODE ARRHYTHMIAS

When the heart functions normally, the sinoatrial (SA) node (also called the *sinus node*) acts as the primary pacemaker. The SA node assumes this role because its automatic firing rate exceeds that of the heart's other pacemakers. In an adult at rest, the SA node has an inherent firing rate of 60 to 100 times per minute.

In about 55% of people, the SA node's blood supply comes from the right coronary artery, and in about 45% of people, it comes from the left circumflex artery. The autonomic nervous system (ANS) richly innervates the SA node through the vagal nerve, a parasympathetic nerve, and several sympathetic nerves. Stimulation of the vagus nerve decreases the SA node's firing rate, and stimulation of the sympathetic system increases it.

ANS influences, or changes in the automaticity of the SA node or in its blood supply, may all lead to SA node arrhythmias. This chapter will help you identify SA node arrhythmias on an electrocardiogram (ECG). It will also help you to determine the causes, significance, signs and symptoms, treatment, and interventions associated with each arrhythmia.

The eight-step method to analyzing the ECG strip will be used for each of the following arrhythmias.

Sinus arrhythmia

In sinus arrhythmia, the rate stays within normal limits but the rhythm is irregular and corresponds to the respiratory cycle, accelerating with inspiration and slowing with expiration. Sinus arrhythmia can occur normally in athletes, children, and older adults, but it rarely occurs in infants. Conditions unrelated to respiration that may also produce sinus arrhythmia include:
● heart disease
● increased intracranial pressure (ICP)
● inferior wall myocardial infarction (MI)
● old age
● use of certain drugs, such as digoxin and morphine.

CAUSES
Sinus arrhythmia, the heart's normal response to breathing, is caused by an inhibition of reflex vagal activity (tone). During inspiration, an increase in the flow of blood back to the heart

RECOGNIZING SINUS ARRHYTHMIA

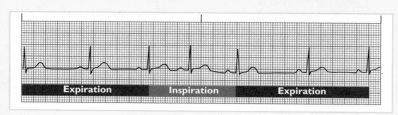

RHYTHM
◆ Irregular
◆ Corresponds to the respiratory cycle
◆ P-P interval and R-R interval shorter during inspiration; longer during expiration
◆ Difference between the longest and the shortest P-P interval exceeds 0.12 seconds

RATE
◆ Usually within normal limits (60 to 100 beats/minute); rate may be less than 60 beats/minute
◆ Varies with respiration
◆ Increases during inspiration
◆ Decreases during expiration

P WAVE
◆ Normal size
◆ Normal configuration

PR INTERVAL
◆ May vary slightly
◆ Within normal limits

QRS COMPLEX
◆ Preceded by P wave
◆ Normal configuration

T WAVE
◆ Normal size
◆ Normal configuration

QT INTERVAL
◆ May vary slightly
◆ Usually within normal limits

OTHER
◆ Phasic slowing and quickening

reduces vagal tone, which increases the heart rate. ECG complexes fall closer together, which shortens the P-P interval. During expiration, venous return decreases, which in turn increases vagal tone, slows the heart rate, and lengthens the P-P interval. (See *Recognizing sinus arrhythmia*.)

CLINICAL SIGNIFICANCE
Sinus arrhythmia usually isn't significant and produces no symptoms. A marked variation in P-P intervals in an elderly adult, however, may indicate sick sinus syndrome—a related, potentially more serious phenomenon.

SIGNS AND SYMPTOMS
The patient may exhibit peripheral pulse rate increases during inspiration and decreases during expiration. Sinus arrhythmia is easier to detect when the heart rate is slow; it may disappear when the heart rate increases, as with exercise.

If the arrhythmia is caused by an underlying condition, you may note signs and symptoms of that condition. Marked sinus arrhythmia may cause dizziness or syncope in some cases.

TREATMENT
Unless the patient is symptomatic, treatment usually isn't necessary. If

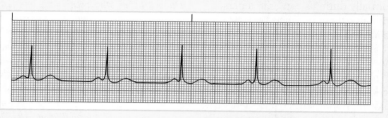

RECOGNIZING SINUS BRADYCARDIA

RHYTHM
◆ Regular

RATE
◆ Less than 60 beats/minute

P WAVE
◆ Normal size
◆ Normal configuration
◆ P wave before each QRS complex

PR INTERVAL
◆ Within normal limits
◆ Constant

QRS COMPLEX
◆ Normal duration
◆ Normal configuration

T WAVE
◆ Normal size
◆ Normal configuration

QT INTERVAL
◆ Within normal limits
◆ Possibly prolonged

OTHER
◆ None

sinus arrhythmia is unrelated to respirations, the underlying cause may require treatment.

NURSING INTERVENTIONS
When caring for a patient with sinus arrhythmia take these actions:
● Monitor the heart rhythm during respiration to determine whether the arrhythmia coincides with the respiratory cycle.
● Check the rhythm carefully to avoid an inaccurate interpretation of the waveform.
● If induced by drugs (such as morphine sulfate or other sedatives), notify the practitioner, who will decide whether to continue the drugs.

Alert *If sinus arrhythmia develops suddenly in a patient taking digoxin,* *notify the practitioner. The patient may be experiencing digoxin toxicity.*

Sinus bradycardia

Sinus bradycardia is characterized by a sinus rate below 60 beats/minute and a regular rhythm. All impulses originate in the SA node. This arrhythmia's significance depends on the symptoms and the underlying cause. (See *Recognizing sinus bradycardia.*)

CAUSES
Sinus bradycardia usually occurs as the normal response to a reduced demand for blood flow. In this case, vagal stimulation increases and sympathetic stimulation decreases. As a result, automaticity (the tendency of

cells to initiate their own impulses) in the SA node diminishes. It may occur normally during sleep or in a person with a well-conditioned heart, such as an athlete.

Sinus bradycardia may be caused by:

- noncardiac disorders, such as hyperkalemia, increased ICP, hypothyroidism, hypothermia, and glaucoma
- conditions that produce excess vagal stimulation or decreased sympathetic stimulation, such as sleep, deep relaxation, the Valsalva maneuver, carotid sinus massage, and vomiting
- cardiac diseases, such as SA node disease, cardiomyopathy, myocarditis, myocardial ischemia, and heart block; also can occur immediately after an inferior wall MI that involves the right coronary artery, which supplies blood to the SA node.
- certain drugs, especially beta blockers; digoxin; calcium-channel blockers; lithium; and antiarrhythmics, such as sotalol, amiodarone, propafenone, and quinidine.

CLINICAL SIGNIFICANCE

The significance of sinus bradycardia depends on how low the rate is and whether the patient is symptomatic. For example, most adults can tolerate a sinus bradycardia of 45 to 59 beats/minute but are less tolerant of a rate lower than 45 beats/minute.

Usually, sinus bradycardia is asymptomatic and insignificant. Many athletes develop sinus bradycardia because their well-conditioned hearts can maintain a normal stroke volume with less-than-normal effort. Sinus bradycardia also occurs normally during sleep as a result of circadian variations in heart rate.

Alert If sinus bradycardia causes symptoms, prompt attention is critical. The heart of a patient with underlying cardiac disease may be unable to compensate for a drop in rate by increasing its stroke volume. The resulting drop in cardiac output produces signs and symptoms, such as hypotension and dizziness. Bradycardia also may predispose some patients to more serious arrhythmias, such as ventricular tachycardia and ventricular fibrillation.

In a patient who has had an acute inferior wall MI, sinus bradycardia is considered a favorable prognostic sign, unless it's accompanied by hypotension. Because sinus bradycardia rarely affects children, it's considered a poor prognostic indicator in this age group.

SIGNS AND SYMPTOMS

The patient will have a pulse rate of less than 60 beats/minute, with a regular rhythm. As long as he's able to compensate for the decreased cardiac output, he'll probably not develop symptoms. If compensatory mechanisms fail, however, signs and symptoms of declining cardiac output usually appear, including:

- altered mental status
- blurred vision
- chest pain
- cool, clammy skin
- crackles, dyspnea, and an S_3 heart sound, indicating heart failure
- dizziness
- hypotension
- syncope.

Palpitations and pulse irregularities may occur if the patient experiences ectopy such as premature atrial, junctional, or ventricular contractions. This is because the SA node's increased relative refractory period permits ectopic firing. Bradycardia-induced syncope (Stokes-Adams attack) also may occur.

TREATMENT

If the patient is asymptomatic and his vital signs are stable, treatment generally isn't necessary. If the patient has symptoms, treatment aims to identify and correct the underlying cause. (See *Bradycardia,* page 262.)

NURSING INTERVENTIONS

When caring for a patient with sinus bradycardia take these actions:
- Observe the patient and monitor the progression and duration of the bradycardia.
- Evaluate the patient's tolerance of the rhythm at rest and with activity.
- Review the patient's drug regimen and check with the practitioner about stopping drugs that may be depressing the SA node, such as digoxin, beta blockers, or calcium-channel blockers.
- Prepare the patient for treatments, such as drug administration (atropine, dopamine, epinephrine) or temporary or permanent pacemaker insertion.
- Administer drugs such as atropine, epinephrine, or dobutamine while awaiting a pacemaker, or if pacing is ineffective.

Alert *Keep in mind that a patient with a transplanted heart won't respond to atropine and may require pacing for emergency treatment.*

Sinus tachycardia

Sinus tachycardia is an acceleration of the firing of the SA node beyond its normal discharge rate. Sinus tachycardia in an adult is characterized by a sinus rate of more than 100 beats/minute. The rate rarely exceeds 180 beats/minute except during strenuous exercise; the maximum rate achievable with exercise decreases with age. (See *Recognizing sinus tachycardia,* page 54.)

CAUSES

Sinus tachycardia may be a normal response to exercise, pain, stress, fever, or strong emotions, such as fear and anxiety. Other causes of sinus tachycardia include:
- cardiac conditions, such as heart failure, cardiogenic shock, and pericarditis
- drugs, such as atropine, isoproterenol, aminophylline, dopamine, dobutamine, epinephrine, alcohol, caffeine, nicotine, and amphetamines
- other conditions, such as shock, anemia, respiratory distress, pulmonary embolism, sepsis, and hyperthyroidism, where the increased heart rate serves as a compensatory mechanism.

CLINICAL SIGNIFICANCE

The significance of sinus tachycardia depends on the underlying cause. The arrhythmia may be the body's response to exercise or strong emotional states, and may be of no clinical significance. It also may occur with hypovolemia, hemorrhage, or pain. When the stimulus for the tachycardia is removed, the arrhythmia generally resolves spontaneously.

Although sinus tachycardia commonly occurs without serious adverse effects, persistent sinus tachycardia can also be serious, especially if it occurs in the setting of an acute MI. Tachycardia can lower cardiac output by reducing ventricular filling time and stroke volume. Normally, ventricular volume reaches 120 to 130 ml during diastole. In tachycardia, decreased ventricular volume leads to

RECOGNIZING SINUS TACHYCARDIA

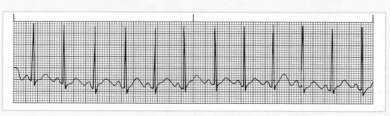

RHYTHM
◆ Regular

RATE
◆ Greater than 100 beats/minute

P WAVE
◆ Normal size
◆ Normal configuration
◆ May increase in amplitude
◆ Precedes each QRS complex
◆ As heart rate increases, possibly superimposed on preceding T wave and difficult to identify

PR INTERVAL
◆ Within normal limits
◆ Constant

QRS COMPLEX
◆ Normal duration
◆ Normal configuration

T WAVE
◆ Normal size
◆ Normal configuration

QT INTERVAL
◆ Within normal limits
◆ Commonly shortened

OTHER
◆ None

decreased cardiac output with subsequent hypotension and decreased peripheral perfusion.

Tachycardia worsens myocardial ischemia by increasing the heart's demand for oxygen and reducing the duration of diastole, the period of greatest coronary blood flow.

An increase in heart rate also can be detrimental for patients with obstructive types of heart conditions, such as aortic stenosis and hypertrophic cardiomyopathy. Persistent tachycardia also may signal impending heart failure or cardiogenic shock. Sinus tachycardia also can cause angina in patients with coronary artery disease.

SIGNS AND SYMPTOMS

The patient will have a peripheral pulse rate above 100 beats/minute, but with a regular rhythm. Usually, he'll be asymptomatic. However, if his cardiac output falls and compensatory mechanisms fail, he may experience:
● anxiety or nervousness
● blurred vision
● chest pain and palpitations
● hypotension
● syncope.

If heart failure develops, he may exhibit crackles, an extra heart sound (S$_3$), and jugular vein distention.

TREATMENT

When treating the asymptomatic patient, you must determine the cause of the tachycardia. The focus of treatment in the symptomatic patient with sinus tachycardia is to maintain adequate cardiac output and tissue perfusion and to identify and correct the underlying cause. For example, if the tachycardia is caused by hemorrhage, treatment includes stopping the bleeding and replacing blood and fluid losses.

If tachycardia leads to cardiac ischemia, treatment may include giving drugs to slow the heart rate. The most commonly used drugs include beta blockers, such as metoprolol and atenolol, and calcium-channel blockers such as verapamil.

NURSING INTERVENTIONS

When caring for a patient with sinus tachycardia take these actions:
● Check the patient's drug history. Over-the-counter sympathomimetics, which mimic the effects of the sympathetic nervous system, may contribute to the sinus tachycardia. Sympathomimetics may be contained in nose drops and cold formulas.
● Ask the patient about his use of caffeine, nicotine, and alcohol, each of which can trigger tachycardia. Advise him to avoid these substances.
● Ask the patient about his use of illicit drugs, such as cocaine and amphetamines, which also can cause tachycardia.
● Assess the patient for signs and symptoms of angina and heart failure.
● Monitor intake and output, and check the patient's weight daily.
● Check the patient's level of consciousness to assess cerebral perfusion.

● Provide a calm environment. Help to reduce the patient's fear and anxiety, which can aggravate his arrhythmia.
● Teach the patient about procedures and treatments, including relaxation techniques.

Alert *Tachycardia is frequently the first sign of a pulmonary embolism. Stay alert to this possibility, especially if your patient has predisposing risk factors for thrombotic emboli. Be aware that a sudden onset of sinus tachycardia after an MI may signal extension of the infarction. Notify the practitioner promptly.*

Sinus arrest and SA exit block

Although sinus arrest and SA exit block (sometimes called *sinus exit block*) are two separate arrhythmias with different etiologies, they're discussed together because distinguishing the two is often difficult. Also, there's no difference in their clinical significance and treatment.

In sinus arrest, the normal sinus rhythm is interrupted by an occasional, prolonged failure of the SA node to initiate an impulse. Therefore, sinus arrest is caused by episodes of failure in the automaticity or impulse formation of the SA node. The atria aren't stimulated, and an entire PQRST complex is missing from the ECG strip. Except for this missing complex, or pause, the ECG usually remains normal. When one or two impulses aren't formed, it's called a sinus pause; when three or more impulses aren't formed, it's called a sinus arrest. (See *Recognizing sinus arrest,* page 56.)

In SA exit block, the SA node discharges at regular intervals, but some

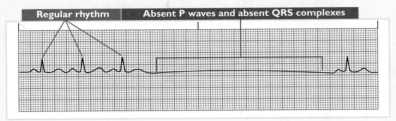

RECOGNIZING SINUS ARREST

| Regular rhythm | Absent P waves and absent QRS complexes |

RHYTHM
◆ Regular except during arrest (irregular as a result of missing complexes)

RATE
◆ Usually within normal limits (60 to 100 beats/minute) before arrest
◆ Length or frequency of pause may cause bradycardia

P WAVE
◆ Periodically absent, with entire PQRST complexes missing
◆ When present, normal size and configuration
◆ Precedes each QRS complex

PR INTERVAL
◆ Within normal limits when a P wave is present
◆ Constant when a P wave is present

QRS COMPLEX
◆ Normal duration
◆ Normal configuration
◆ Absent during arrest

T WAVE
◆ Normal size
◆ Normal configuration
◆ Absent during arrest

QT INTERVAL
◆ Within normal limits
◆ Absent during arrest

OTHER
◆ The pause isn't a multiple of the underlying P-P intervals

impulses are delayed or blocked from reaching the atria, resulting in long sinus pauses. Blocks result from failure to conduct impulses, while sinus arrest is caused by a failure to form impulses in the SA node. Both arrhythmias cause atrial activity to stop. In sinus arrest, the pause often ends with a junctional escape beat. In SA exit block, the pause occurs for an indefinite period and ends with a sinus rhythm. (See *Recognizing sinoatrial exit block*.)

CAUSES
Causes of sinus arrest and SA exit block include:
● acute infection
● digoxin, quinidine, procainamide, and salicylate toxicity
● cardiac disorders, such as coronary artery disease, acute myocarditis, cardiomyopathy, hypertensive heart disease, and acute inferior wall MI
● excessive doses of beta blockers such as metoprolol and propranolol
● increased vagal tone, such as with the Valsalva maneuver, carotid sinus massage, or vomiting

RECOGNIZING SINOATRIAL EXIT BLOCK

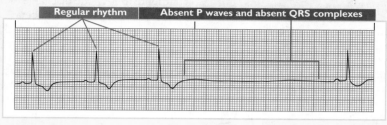

| Regular rhythm | Absent P waves and absent QRS complexes |

RHYTHM
◆ Regular except during pause (irregular as result of pause)

RATE
◆ Usually within normal limits (60 to 100 beats/minute) before pause
◆ Length or frequency of pause may cause bradycardia

P WAVE
◆ Periodically absent, with entire PQRST complexes missing
◆ When present, normal size and configuration and precedes each QRS complex

PR INTERVAL
◆ Within normal limits
◆ Constant when a P wave is present

QRS COMPLEX
◆ Normal duration
◆ Normal configuration
◆ Absent during a pause

T WAVE
◆ Normal size
◆ Normal configuration
◆ Absent during a pause

QT INTERVAL
◆ Within normal limits
◆ Absent during a pause

OTHER
◆ The pause is a multiple of the underlying P-P interval

● SA node disease, such as fibrosis and idiopathic degeneration
● sick sinus syndrome.

CLINICAL SIGNIFICANCE

The significance of these two arrhythmias depends on the patient's symptoms. If the pauses are short and infrequent, the patient will most likely be asymptomatic and will not require treatment. He may have a normal sinus rhythm for days or weeks between episodes of sinus arrest or SA exit block, and he may be totally unaware of the arrhythmia. Pauses of 2 or 3 seconds normally occur in healthy adults during sleep, and occasionally in patients with increased vagal tone or hypersensitive carotid sinus disease.

If either of the arrhythmias is frequent or prolonged, however, the patient will most likely experience symptoms related to low cardiac output. The arrhythmias can produce syncope or near-syncopal episodes usually within 7 seconds of asystole.

Alert *During a prolonged pause, the patient may fall and injure himself. Other situations are potentially just as serious. For example, a symptomatic arrhythmia that occurs while the patient is driving a car could cause a fatal accident. Extremely slow rates can also produce other arrhythmias.*

Differentiation criteria

To differentiate between these two rhythms, compare the length of the pause with the underlying P-P or R-R interval. If the underlying rhythm is regular, determine if the rhythm resumes on time after the pause. With SA exit block, because the regularity of the SA node discharge is blocked, not interrupted, the underlying rhythm will resume on time after the pause. In addition, the length of the pause will be a multiple of the underlying P-P or R-R interval.

In sinus arrest, the timing of the SA node discharge is interrupted by the failure of the SA node to initiate an impulse. As a result, the underlying rhythm doesn't resume on time after the pause, and the length of the pause is not a multiple of the previous R-R intervals.

SIGNS AND SYMPTOMS

You won't be able to detect a pulse or heart sounds when sinus arrest or SA exit block occurs. Short pauses usually produce no symptoms. Recurrent or prolonged pauses may cause signs of decreased cardiac output, such as:

- altered mental status
- cool, clammy skin
- dizziness or blurred vision
- low blood pressure
- syncopal episodes.

TREATMENT

An asymptomatic patient needs no treatment. Symptomatic patients are treated following the guidelines for patients with symptomatic bradycardia. (See *Bradycardia, page 262.*) Treatment also will focus on the cause

of the sinus arrest or SA exit block. This may involve stopping drugs that contribute to SA node discharge or conduction, such as digoxin, beta blockers, and calcium-channel blockers.

NURSING INTERVENTIONS

When caring for a patient with sinus arrest or SA exit block take these actions:

- Monitor the heart rhythm.
- Observe the circumstances under which the pauses occur. Both sinus arrest and SA exit block may be insignificant if detected while the patient is sleeping.
- Protect the patient from injury, such as a fall, which may result from a syncopal or near-syncopal pause.
- If the pauses are recurrent, assess the patient for evidence of decreased cardiac output, such as altered mental status, low blood pressure, and cool, clammy skin.
- Document the patient's vital signs and how he feels during pauses as well as the activities in which he was involved at the time.
- Assess for a progression of the arrhythmia. Notify the practitioner immediately if the patient becomes unstable.
- Be alert for signs of digoxin, quinidine, or procainamide toxicity. Obtain digoxin and electrolyte levels.

Sick sinus syndrome

Also known as *SA syndrome, sinus nodal dysfunction,* and *Stokes-Adams syndrome,* sick sinus syndrome (SSS) refers to a wide spectrum of SA node arrhythmias. This syndrome is caused by disturbances in the way impulses are generated or in the ability to conduct impulses to the atria. These disturbances may be either intrinsic or mediated by the ANS.

SSS usually shows up as bradycardia, with episodes of sinus arrest and SA block interspersed with sudden, brief periods of rapid atrial fibrillation. Patients are also prone to paroxysms of other atrial tachyarrhythmias, such as atrial flutter and ectopic atrial tachycardia, a condition sometimes referred to as bradycardia-tachycardia (or brady-tachy) syndrome.

Most patients with SSS are older than age 60, but anyone can develop the arrhythmia. It's rare in children except after open-heart surgery that results in SA node damage. The arrhythmia affects men and women equally. The onset is progressive, insidious, and chronic. (See *Recognizing sick sinus syndrome*.)

CAUSES

SSS results either from a dysfunction of the SA node's automaticity or from abnormal conduction or blockages of impulses from the nodal region. These conditions, in turn, stem from a degeneration of the area's ANS and partial destruction of the SA node, as may occur with an interrupted blood supply after an inferior wall MI.

In addition, certain conditions can affect the atrial wall surrounding the SA node and cause exit blocks.

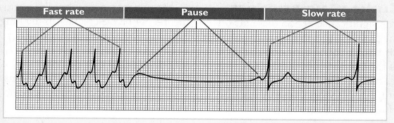

RECOGNIZING SICK SINUS SYNDROME

| Fast rate | Pause | Slow rate |

RHYTHM
◆ Irregular with sinus pauses

RATE
◆ Fast, slow, or alternating
◆ Abrupt rate changes
◆ Interrupted by a long sinus pause

P WAVE
◆ Varies with rhythm changes
◆ May be normal size and configuration
◆ May be absent
◆ Usually precedes each QRS complex

PR INTERVAL
◆ Usually within normal limits
◆ Varies with rhythm changes

QRS COMPLEX
◆ Duration within normal limits
◆ Varies with rhythm changes
◆ Normal configuration

T WAVE
◆ Normal size
◆ Normal configuration

QT INTERVAL
◆ Usually within normal limits
◆ Varies with rhythm changes

OTHER
◆ Usually more than one arrhythmia on a 6-second strip

Conditions that cause inflammation or degeneration of atrial tissue can also lead to SSS. However, in many patients the exact cause is never identified.

Causes of SSS include:

- autonomic disturbances that affect autonomic innervation, such as hypervagotonia or degeneration of the autonomic system
- cardioactive drugs, such as digoxin, beta blockers, and calcium-channel blockers
- conditions that cause fibrosis of the SA node, such as increased age, atherosclerotic heart disease, hypertension, ischemia, MI, and cardiomyopathy
- trauma to the SA node caused by open-heart surgery (especially valvular surgery), pericarditis, or rheumatic heart disease.

CLINICAL SIGNIFICANCE

The significance of SSS depends on the patient's age, the presence of other diseases, and the type and duration of the specific arrhythmias that occur. If atrial fibrillation is involved, the prognosis is worse, mainly because of the risk of thromboembolic complications.

If prolonged pauses are involved with SSS, syncope may occur. The length of a pause needed to cause syncope varies with the patient's age, posture at the time, and cerebrovascular status. Any pause that lasts 2 or 3 seconds or more is considered significant.

It's important to determine whether the patient experiences symptoms while the disturbance occurs. Because the syndrome is progressive and chronic, a symptomatic patient will need lifelong treatment. In addition, thromboembolism may develop as a complication of SSS, possibly resulting in stroke or peripheral embolization.

SIGNS AND SYMPTOMS

The patient's pulse rate may be fast, slow, or normal, and the rhythm may be regular or irregular. You can usually detect an irregularity on the monitor or when palpating the pulse, which may feel at first inappropriately slow, and then rapid.

If you monitor the patient's heart rate during exertion, you may observe inappropriate responses to exercise, such as:

- atrial fibrillation
- atrial flutter
- brady-tachy syndrome
- failure of the heart rate to increase
- SA block
- sinus arrest on the monitor.

Other assessment findings depend on the patient's condition. For example, he may have crackles in the lungs, S_3, or a dilated and displaced left ventricular apical impulse if he has underlying cardiomyopathy.

The patient also may show signs and symptoms of decreased cardiac output, such as:

- blurred vision
- fatigue
- hypotension
- syncope (a common symptom with this arrhythmia).

Alert When caring for a patient with SSS, be alert for signs and symptoms of thromboembolism, especially if the patient experiences atrial fibrillation. Blood clots or thrombi forming in the heart can dislodge and travel through the bloodstream, resulting in decreased blood supply to the lungs, heart, brain, kidneys, intestines, or other organs. Assess the patient for neurologic changes, such as confusion, vision disturbances, weakness, chest pain, dyspnea, tachypnea, tachycardia, and acute on-

set of pain. Early recognition enables prompt treatment.

TREATMENT

As with other SA node arrhythmias, no treatment is generally necessary if the patient is asymptomatic. If the patient is symptomatic, however, treatment aims to relieve signs and symptoms and correct the underlying cause of the arrhythmia.

Atropine or epinephrine may be given initially for symptomatic bradycardia. (See *Bradycardia,* page 262.) A temporary pacemaker may be required until the underlying disorder resolves. Tachyarrhythmias may be treated with antiarrhythmics, such as metoprolol and digoxin. Unfortunately, drugs used to suppress tachyarrhythmias may worsen underlying SA node disease and bradyarrhythmias.

The patient may need anticoagulants if he develops sudden bursts, or paroxysms, of atrial fibrillation. The anticoagulants help prevent thromboembolism and stroke, which are complications of the condition.

NURSING INTERVENTIONS

When caring for a patient with SSS take these actions:

- Monitor and document all arrhythmias, as well as signs or symptoms.
- Note changes in heart rate and rhythm related to changes in the patient's level of activity.
- Look for signs and symptoms of thromboembolism, especially if the patient experiences atrial fibrillation. Blood clots or thrombi forming in the heart can dislodge and travel through the bloodstream, decreasing blood supply to the lungs, heart, brain, kidneys, intestines, or other organs.

- Assess the patient for neurologic changes, such as confusion, vision disturbances, weakness, chest pain, dyspnea, tachypnea, tachycardia, and acute onset of pain. Early recognition allows for prompt treatment.
- Watch the patient carefully after starting beta and calcium-channel blockers, or other antiarrhythmics.
- Prepare the patient for possible treatment interventions, such as anticoagulant therapy and pacemaker insertion.

5

ATRIAL ARRHYTHMIAS

Atrial arrhythmias, the most common cardiac rhythm disturbances, result from impulses that originate in the atrial tissue outside of the sinoatrial (SA) node. These arrhythmias can affect ventricular filling time and diminish *atrial kick*, which is the complete filling of the ventricles during atrial systole. Atrial kick accounts for 15% to 25% of cardiac output in healthy adults and up to 50% of cardiac output in those with decreased ventricular compliance. This loss of atrial kick may greatly decrease cardiac output and cause decreased perfusion in some patients.

Atrial arrhythmias are probably caused by these three mechanisms: altered automaticity, reentry, and afterdepolarization.

Altered automaticity

The term "automaticity" refers to the ability of cardiac cells to initiate electric impulses spontaneously. An increase in the automaticity of the atrial fibers can trigger abnormal impulses. Causes of increased automaticity include extracellular factors, such as hypoxia, hypocalcemia, and digoxin toxicity, as well as conditions in which the function of the heart's normal pacemaker (the SA node) is diminished. For example, increased vagal tone or hypokalemia can increase the refractory period of the SA node and allow atrial fibers to initiate impulses.

Reentry

In reentry, an impulse is delayed along a slow conduction pathway. Despite the delay, the impulse remains active enough to produce another impulse during myocardial repolarization, resulting in an abnormal continuous circuit. Reentry may occur with coronary artery disease (CAD), cardiomyopathy, or myocardial infarction (MI) and is the most common mechanism in atrial arrhythmias.

Afterdepolarization

Afterdepolarization can occur as a result of cell injury, digoxin toxicity, and other conditions. An injured cell sometimes only partially repolarizes. Partial repolarization can lead to repetitive ectopic firing (called "triggered activity"). The depolarization produced by triggered activity, known as afterdepolarization, can lead to atrial or ventricular tachycardia.

This chapter will help you identify atrial arrhythmias, including premature atrial contractions (PACs), atrial tachycardia, atrial flutter, atrial fibrillation, Ashman's phenomenon, and wandering pacemaker. The chapter reviews causes, clinical significance, electrocardiogram (ECG) characteristics, and signs and symptoms of each arrhythmia as well as treatments for these arrhythmias.

Premature atrial contractions

PACs originate in the atria, outside the SA node. They arise from either a single ectopic focus or from multiple atrial foci that supersede the SA node as pacemaker for one or more beats. PACs are generally caused by enhanced automaticity in the atrial tissue. (See *Identifying premature atrial contractions,* page 64.)

PACs may be conducted or non-conducted (blocked) through the atrioventricular (AV) node and the rest of the heart, depending on the status of the AV and intraventricular conduction system. If the atrial ectopic pacemaker discharges too early after the preceding QRS complex, the AV junction or bundle branches may still be refractory from conducting the previous electric impulse. If they're still refractory, they may not be sufficiently repolarized to conduct the premature electric impulse into the ventricles normally.

When a PAC is conducted, ventricular conduction is usually normal. Nonconducted, or blocked, PACs aren't followed by a QRS complex. At times it may be difficult to distinguish nonconducted PACs from SA block. (See *Distinguishing nonconducted PACs from SA block,* page 65.)

CAUSES
Alcohol, cigarettes, anxiety, fatigue, caffeine, fever, and infectious diseases can trigger PACs, which commonly occur in a normal heart. Elimination or control of those factors can usually correct the arrhythmia.

PACs may be associated with:
- acute respiratory failure
- certain electrolyte imbalances
- chronic pulmonary disease
- coronary or valvular heart disease
- digoxin toxicity
- hyperthyroidism
- hypoxia.

PACs may be caused by drugs that prolong the absolute refractory period of the SA node, including quinidine and procainamide. Endogenous catecholamine release during episodes of pain or anxiety may also cause PACs.

CLINICAL SIGNIFICANCE
PACs are rarely dangerous in patients who don't have heart disease; they often cause no symptoms and go unrecognized for years. Patients may perceive PACs as palpitations or skipped beats.

However, in patients with heart disease, PACs may lead to more serious arrhythmias, such as atrial fibrillation or atrial flutter.

Alert *In a patient with acute MI, PACs can serve as an early sign of heart failure or electrolyte imbalance.*

SIGNS AND SYMPTOMS
The patient may have an irregular peripheral or apical pulse rhythm when the PACs occur. Otherwise, the pulse rhythm and rate will reflect the underlying rhythm. Patients may complain of palpitations, skipped beats, or a fluttering sensation. In a patient with heart disease, signs and

IDENTIFYING PREMATURE ATRIAL CONTRACTIONS

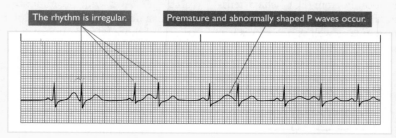

The rhythm is irregular.

Premature and abnormally shaped P waves occur.

RHYTHM
♦ Atrial: Irregular
♦ Ventricular: Irregular
♦ Underlying: Possibly regular

RATE
♦ Atrial and ventricular: Vary with underlying rhythm

P WAVE
♦ Premature
♦ Abnormal configuration compared to a sinus P wave
♦ If varying configurations, multiple ectopic sites
♦ May be hidden in preceding T wave

PR INTERVAL
♦ Usually within normal limits
♦ May be shortened or slightly prolonged for the ectopic beat, depending on the origin of ectopic focus

QRS COMPLEX
♦ Conducted: Duration and configuration usually normal
♦ Nonconducted: No QRS complex follows premature atrial contraction (PAC)

T WAVE
♦ Usually normal
♦ May be distorted if P wave is hidden in T wave

QT INTERVAL
♦ Usually within normal limits

OTHER
♦ May be a single beat
♦ May be bigeminal (every other beat premature)
♦ May be trigeminal (every third beat premature)
♦ May be quadrigeminal (every fourth beat premature)
♦ May occur in couplets (pairs)
♦ Three or more PACs in a row indicating atrial tachycardia

---

symptoms of decreased cardiac output, such as hypotension and syncope, may occur.

TREATMENT
Most asymptomatic patients don't need treatment. If the patient is symptomatic, treatment may focus on eliminating the cause, such as caffeine and alcohol. People with frequent PACs may be treated with drugs that prolong the refractory period of the atria. Those drugs include digoxin, as well as calcium-channel and beta blockers.

NURSING INTERVENTIONS
● Assess the patient to help determine factors that trigger ectopic beats.

Look-alikes

DISTINGUISHING NONCONDUCTED PACs FROM SA BLOCK

To differentiate nonconducted premature atrial contractions (PACs) from sinoatrial (SA) block, check the following:

◆ Whenever you see a pause in a rhythm, look carefully for a nonconducted P wave, which may occur before, during, or just after the T wave preceding the pause.

◆ Compare T waves that precede a pause with the other T waves in the rhythm strip, and look for a distortion of the slope of the T wave or a difference in its height or shape. These are clues showing you where the nonconducted P wave may be hidden.

◆ If you find a P wave in the pause, check to see whether it's premature or if it occurs earlier than subsequent sinus P waves. If it's premature (see shaded area below, top), you can be certain it's a nonconducted PAC.

◆ If there's no P wave in the pause or T wave (see shaded area below, bottom), the rhythm is SA block.

Nonconducted PAC

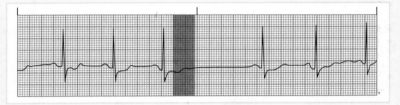

SA block

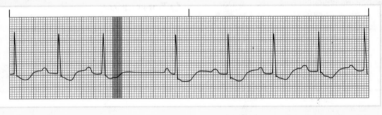

● If the patient has ischemic or valvular heart disease, monitor for signs and symptoms of heart failure, electrolyte imbalance, and more severe atrial arrhythmias.

● Teach patient to correct or avoid underlying causes. For example, the patient might need to avoid caffeine or learn stress reduction techniques to lessen anxiety.

Atrial tachycardia

Atrial tachycardia is a supraventricular tachycardia, which means that the impulses driving the rapid rhythm originate above the ventricles. Atrial tachycardia has an atrial rate from 150 to 250 beats/minute. The rapid rate shortens diastole, resulting in a loss of

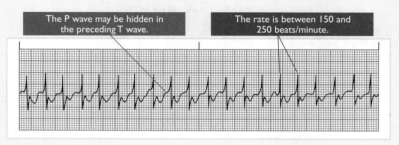

IDENTIFYING ATRIAL TACHYCARDIA

The P wave may be hidden in the preceding T wave.

The rate is between 150 and 250 beats/minute.

RHYTHM
◆ Atrial: Usually regular
◆ Ventricular: Regular or irregular depending on atrioventricular (AV) conduction ratio and type of atrial tachycardia

RATE
◆ Atrial: Three or more consecutive ectopic atrial beats at 150 to 250 beats/minute; rarely exceeds 250 beats/minute
◆ Ventricular: Varies, depending on AV-conduction ratio

P WAVE
◆ Deviates from normal appearance
◆ May be hidden in preceding T wave
◆ If visible, usually upright and preceding each QRS complex

PR INTERVAL
◆ Within normal limits, or may be difficult to measure if P wave can't be distinguished from preceding T wave

QRS COMPLEX
◆ Usually normal duration and configuration
◆ May be abnormal if impulses conducted abnormally through ventricles

T WAVE
◆ Usually visible
◆ May be distorted by P wave
◆ May be inverted if ischemia is present

QT INTERVAL
◆ Usually within normal limits
◆ May be shorter because of rapid rate

OTHER
◆ None

atrial kick, reduced cardiac output, reduced coronary perfusion, and the potential for myocardial ischemia. (See *Identifying atrial tachycardia*.)

Three forms of atrial tachycardia are discussed here. They include:
● atrial tachycardia with block
● multifocal atrial tachycardia (MAT), also known as *chaotic atrial tachycardia*
● paroxysmal atrial tachycardia (PAT).

In atrial tachycardia with block, not all atrial impulses are conducted through to the ventricles. In MAT, the tachycardia originates from multiple atrial foci. PAT is generally a transient event in which the tachycardia appears and disappears suddenly. (See *Identifying types of atrial tachycardia*.)

CAUSES
Atrial tachycardia can occur in patients with a normal heart. In those

IDENTIFYING TYPES OF ATRIAL TACHYCARDIA

CHARACTERISTICS OF ATRIAL TACHYCARDIA WITH BLOCK

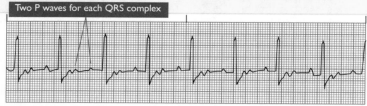

Two P waves for each QRS complex

◆ *Rhythm:* atrial—regular; ventricular—regular if block is constant; irregular if block is variable
◆ *Rate:* atrial—150 to 250 beats/minute and a multiple of ventricular rate; ventricular—varies with block
◆ *P wave:* abnormal

◆ *PR interval:* can vary but is usually constant for conducted P waves
◆ *QRS complex:* usually normal
◆ *T wave:* usually distorted
◆ *QT interval:* may be indiscernible
◆ *Other:* more than one P wave for each QRS complex

CHARACTERISTICS OF MULTIFOCAL ATRIAL TACHYCARDIA

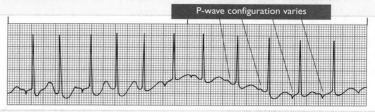

P-wave configuration varies

◆ *Rhythm:* both irregular
◆ *Rate:* atrial—100 to 250 beats/minute; ventricular—100 to 250 beats/minute
◆ *P wave:* configuration varies; usually at least three different P-wave shapes must appear

◆ *PR interval:* varies
◆ *QRS complex:* usually normal, may become aberrant if arrhythmia persists
◆ *T wave:* usually distorted
◆ *QT interval:* may be indiscernible

CHARACTERISTICS OF PAROXYSMAL ATRIAL TACHYCARDIA

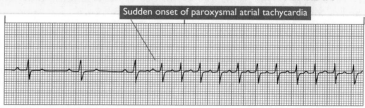

Sudden onset of paroxysmal atrial tachycardia

◆ *Rhythm:* atrial and ventricular—regular
◆ *Rate:* both 150 to 250 beats/minute
◆ *P wave:* abnormal; may not be visible or may be difficult to distinguish from the preceding T wave
◆ *PR interval:* usually within normal limits but may be unmeasurable if the P wave

can't be distinguished from the preceding T wave
◆ *QRS complex:* usually normal, but can be aberrantly conducted
◆ *T wave:* usually distorted
◆ *QT interval:* may be indistinguishable
◆ *Other:* sudden onset, typically initiated by a premature atrial contraction

cases, it's commonly caused by excessive use of caffeine or other stimulants, marijuana, electrolyte imbalance, hypoxia, or physical or psychological stress. Most commonly, though, atrial tachycardia is caused by an ectopic focus in the atria, or primary or secondary cardiac disorders, including:

- cardiomyopathy
- congenital anomalies
- MI
- valvular heart disease
- Wolff-Parkinson-White syndrome.

This rhythm may also be a component of sick sinus syndrome. Other problems resulting in atrial tachycardia include:

- chronic obstructive pulmonary disorder
- cor pulmonale
- digoxin toxicity, the most common cause of atrial tachycardia
- hyperthyroidism
- systemic hypertension.

CLINICAL SIGNIFICANCE

In a healthy person, nonsustained atrial tachycardia is usually benign. The increased ventricular rate that occurs in atrial tachycardia results in decreased ventricular filling time, increased myocardial oxygen consumption, and decreased oxygen supply to the myocardium. Heart failure, myocardial ischemia, and MI can result.

SIGNS AND SYMPTOMS

The patient with atrial tachycardia will have a rapid heart rate. He may complain that his heart suddenly starts to beat faster or that he suddenly feels palpitations. Persistent tachycardia and rapid ventricular rate cause decreased cardiac output, resulting in

hypotension and syncope and dilated cardiomyopathy, if left untreated.

TREATMENT

Treatment depends on the type of tachycardia, the width of the QRS complex, and the stability of the patient's condition. (For specific treatments, see Tachycardia algorithm, page 264.)

The Valsalva maneuver or carotid sinus massage may be used to treat PAT. (See *Understanding carotid sinus massage.*) These maneuvers increase the parasympathetic tone, which results in a slowing of the heart rate. They also allow the SA node to resume function as the primary pacemaker. Older adults may have undiagnosed carotid atherosclerosis and carotid bruits may be absent, even with significant disease. As a result, carotid sinus massage may be inappropriate in late middle-age and older patients.

Alert *Keep in mind that vagal stimulation can cause bradycardia, ventricular arrhythmias, and asystole. If vagal maneuvers are used, make sure resuscitative equipment is readily available.*

Drug therapy (pharmacologic cardioversion) may be used to increase the degree of AV block and decrease ventricular response rate. Appropriate drugs include digoxin and calcium channel blockers and beta-adrenergic blockers. When other treatments fail, or if the patient is unstable, synchronized electric cardioversion may be used.

Atrial overdrive pacing (also called *rapid atrial pacing* or *overdrive suppression*) also may be used to stop the arrhythmia. With this technique, spontaneous depolarization of the ectopic pacemaker is suppressed by a series of

UNDERSTANDING CAROTID SINUS MASSAGE

Carotid sinus massage may be used to interrupt paroxysmal atrial tachycardia. Massaging the carotid sinus stimulates the vagus nerve, which inhibits firing of the sinoatrial (SA) node and slows atrioventricular (AV) node conduction. As a result, the SA node can resume its function as primary pacemaker.

Carotid sinus massage involves a firm massage that lasts no longer than 5 to 10 seconds. The patient's head is turned to the left to massage the right carotid sinus, as illustrated below. Remember never to attempt simultaneous, bilateral massage.

Carotid sinus massage is contraindicated in patients with carotid bruits. Risks of the procedure include decreased heart rate, syncope, sinus arrest, increased degree of AV block, cerebral emboli, cerebrovascular accident, and asystole.

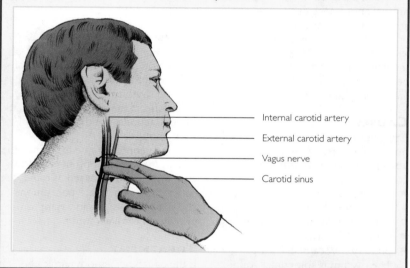

Internal carotid artery

External carotid artery

Vagus nerve

Carotid sinus

paced electric impulses at a rate slightly higher than the intrinsic ectopic atrial rate. The pacemaker cells are depolarized prematurely and, following termination of the paced electric impulses, the SA node resumes its normal role as the pacemaker.

Radiofrequency ablation can also be used to treat PAT. The ectopic focus is mapped during the electrophysiology study, and then the area is ablated. Because MAT commonly occurs in patients with chronic pulmonary disease, the rhythm may not respond to treatment.

NURSING INTERVENTIONS

● Monitor the patient's heart rate and rhythm.

✳ *Best lead* Leads II, V_1, V_6, MCL_1, or MCL_6 are the best choices for monitoring the patient with atrial tachycardia.

● Assess the patient for signs and symptoms of digoxin toxicity and monitor digoxin blood levels.

● Monitor the patient for chest pain, indications of decreased cardiac output, and signs and symptoms of heart failure or myocardial ischemia.

Atrial flutter

Atrial flutter (a supraventricular tachycardia) is characterized by a rapid atrial rate of 200 to 350 beats/minute, although it's generally around 300 beats/minute. Originating in an atrial focus, this rhythm results from a single reentry circuit in the right atria.

On an ECG, the P waves lose their normal appearance due to the rapid atrial rate. The waves blend together in a sawtooth configuration called *flutter waves* (*F waves*). These waves are the hallmark of atrial flutter and are best seen in leads II, III, and V_1. (See *Identifying atrial flutter.*)

Causes

Atrial flutter may be caused by conditions that enlarge atrial tissue and raise atrial pressures. This arrhythmia is commonly found in patients with:
- digoxin toxicity
- hyperthyroidism
- mitral or tricuspid valvular disease
- pericardial disease
- primary myocardial disease.

The rhythm is sometimes found in patients with:
- acute MI
- chronic pulmonary disease
- recent cardiac surgery
- systemic arterial hypoxia.

Atrial flutter rarely occurs in healthy people. However, when it does appear in an apparently healthy person, it may indicate intrinsic heart disease.

Clinical significance

The significance of atrial flutter is determined by the number of impulses conducted through the AV node. That number is expressed as a conduction ratio, such as 2:1 or 4:1, and the resulting ventricular rate. If the ventricular rate is too slow (less than 40 beats/minute) or too fast (greater than 150 beats/minute), cardiac output can be seriously compromised.

Usually, the faster the ventricular rate, the more dangerous the arrhythmia. Rapid ventricular rates reduce ventricular filling time and coronary perfusion, which can cause angina, heart failure, pulmonary edema, hypotension, and syncope.

Signs and symptoms

When caring for a patient with atrial flutter, you may note that the peripheral and apical pulses are normal in rate and rhythm. That's because the pulse reflects the number of ventricular contractions, not the number of atrial impulses.

If the ventricular rate is normal, the patient may be asymptomatic. However, if the ventricular rate is rapid, the patient may experience palpitations and may show signs and symptoms of reduced cardiac output.

Treatment

If the patient is hemodynamically unstable, synchronized electric cardioversion or countershock should be given immediately. Cardioversion delivers an electric current to the heart to correct an arrhythmia and is synchronized to discharge at the peak of the R wave. Atrial flutter is usually easily converted with a low-energy level. This causes immediate depolarization, interrupting reentry circuits and allowing the SA node to resume control as pacemaker.

The focus of treatment for hemodynamically stable patients with atrial flutter includes controlling the rate and converting the rhythm. Specific interventions depend on the patient's

IDENTIFYING ATRIAL FLUTTER

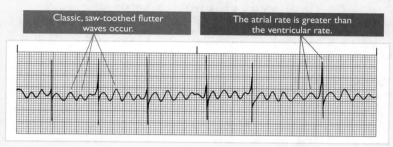

Classic, saw-toothed flutter waves occur.

The atrial rate is greater than the ventricular rate.

RHYTHM
◆ Atrial: Regular
◆ Ventricular: Typically regular; may be irregular because cycles may alternate (depends on atrioventricular [AV] conduction pattern)

RATE
◆ Atrial: 250 to 400 beats/minute
◆ Ventricular: Usually 60 to 150 beats/minute (one-half to one-fourth of atrial rate) but varies depending on degree of AV block
◆ Usually expressed as a ratio (2:1 or 4:1, for example)
◆ Commonly 300 beats/minute atrial and 150 beats/minute ventricular, known as *2:1 block*
◆ Only every second, third, or fourth impulse is conducted to ventricles because the AV node usually won't accept more than 180 impulses/minute
◆ When atrial flutter is first recognized, ventricular rate typically greater than 100 beats/minute

P WAVE
◆ Abnormal
◆ Sawtooth appearance known as *flutter waves* or *F waves*

PR INTERVAL
◆ Not measurable

QRS COMPLEX
◆ Duration: Usually within normal limits
◆ May be widened if flutter waves are buried within the complex

T WAVE
◆ Not identifiable

QT INTERVAL
◆ Not measurable because T wave isn't identifiable

OTHER
◆ Atrial rhythm possibly varying between a fibrillatory line and flutter waves (called *atrial fib-flutter*), with an irregular ventricular response
◆ May be difficult to differentiate atrial flutter from atrial fibrillation

cardiac function, whether preexcitation syndromes are involved, and the duration (less than or more than 48 hours) of the arrhythmia. For example, in atrial flutter with normal cardiac function and duration of rhythm less than 48 hours, direct current (DC) cardioversion may be considered; for duration longer than 48 hours, no DC cardioversion should be considered because it increases the risk of thromboembolism, unless the patient's blood has been adequately anticoagulated.

DISTINGUISHING ATRIAL FLUTTER FROM ATRIAL FIBRILLATION

It isn't uncommon to see atrial flutter with an irregular pattern of impulse conduction to the ventricles. In some leads, this may be confused with atrial fibrillation. Here's how to tell the two arrhythmias apart:

ATRIAL FLUTTER
◆ Look for characteristic abnormal P waves that produce a sawtooth appearance, referred to as *flutter waves*, or *F waves*. These can best be identified in leads II, III, and V_1 on the 12-lead electrocardiogram.
◆ Remember that the atrial rhythm is regular. You should be able to map the flutter waves across the rhythm strip. While some flutter waves may occur within the QRS or T waves, subsequent flutter waves will be visible and occur on time.

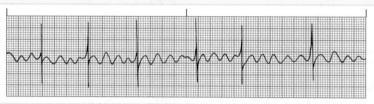

ATRIAL FIBRILLATION
◆ Fibrillatory or *f waves* occur in an irregular pattern, making the atrial rhythm irregular.
◆ If you identify atrial activity that at times looks like flutter waves that seem to be briefly regular, and at other places the rhythm strip contains fibrillatory waves, interpret the rhythm as "atrial fibrillation." Coarse fibrillatory waves may intermittently look like the characteristic sawtooth appearance of flutter waves.

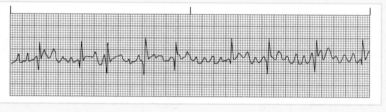

NURSING INTERVENTIONS
● Monitor the patient's heart rate and rhythm. At times it may be difficult to distinguish atrial flutter from atrial fibrillation. (See *Distinguishing atrial flutter from atrial fibrillation*.)

✳ ***Best lead*** *Leads II and III are the best leads for monitoring the patient with atrial flutter.*

● Monitor the patient closely for signs and symptoms of low cardiac output, such as hypotension and changes in mental status.
● Be alert to the effects of digoxin, which depresses the SA node.
● If electric cardioversion is indicated, prepare the patient for I.V. administration of a sedative or anesthetic as ordered. Keep resuscitative equipment at the bedside. Be alert for bradycardia, because cardioversion can decrease the heart rate.

Atrial fibrillation

Atrial fibrillation, sometimes called *AFib*, is defined as chaotic, asynchronous, electric activity in atrial tissue. It's the most common arrhythmia, affecting an estimated 2 million people in the United States. Caused by the firing of multiple reentry circuits in the atria, atrial fibrillation is characterized by the absence of P waves and an irregularly irregular ventricular response.

When a number of ectopic sites in the atria initiate impulses, depolarization can't spread in an organized manner. Because small sections of the atria are depolarized individually, the atrial muscle quivers instead of contracts. On an ECG, uneven baseline fibrillation waves (F waves) appear instead of clearly distinguishable P waves, which may be coarse or fine.

The AV node protects the ventricles from the 350 to 600 erratic atrial impulses that occur each minute by acting as a filter and blocking some of the impulses. The ventricles respond only to impulses conducted through the AV node; hence, the characteristic, wide variation in R-R intervals. When the ventricular response rate is less than 100 beats/minute, atrial fibrillation is considered to be controlled. When the ventricular rate is greater than 100 beats/minute, the rhythm is considered uncontrolled.

As with atrial flutter, atrial fibrillation results in a loss of atrial kick. The rhythm may be sustained or paroxysmal, meaning that it occurs suddenly and ends abruptly. It can either be preceded by or be the result of PACs. (See *Identifying atrial fibrillation,* page 74.)

CAUSES

Atrial fibrillation can occur after cardiothoracic surgery. Other causes of atrial fibrillation include:

- acute MI
- atrial septal defects
- CAD
- cardiomyopathy
- chronic pulmonary disease
- congenital heart defects
- hypertension
- hyperthyroidism
- pericarditis
- rheumatic heart disease
- valvular heart disease (especially mitral valve disease).

The rhythm also may occur in a healthy person who smokes, who drinks coffee or alcohol, or who is tired and stressed. Certain drugs, such as aminophylline and digoxin, may contribute to the development of atrial fibrillation. Endogenous catecholamine released during exercise may also trigger the arrhythmia.

CLINICAL SIGNIFICANCE

The loss of atrial kick from atrial fibrillation can result in the subsequent loss of about 20% of normal end-diastolic volume. Combined with the decreased diastolic filling time associated with a rapid heart rate, cardiac output may be reduced by 50%. In uncontrolled atrial fibrillation, the patient may develop heart failure, myocardial ischemia, or syncope.

Patients with preexisting cardiac disease, such as hypertrophic cardiomyopathy, mitral stenosis, rheumatic heart disease, or those with mitral prosthetic valves, tend to tolerate atrial fibrillation poorly and may develop severe heart failure.

IDENTIFYING ATRIAL FIBRILLATION

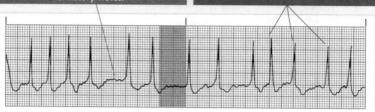

The sinus P wave is replaced by erratic fibrillatory waves.

The rhythm is irregularly irregular.

RHYTHM
◆ Atrial: Irregularly irregular
◆ Ventricular: Irregularly irregular

RATE
◆ Atrial: Almost indiscernible, usually greater than 400 beats/minute; far exceeds ventricular rate because most impulses aren't conducted through the atrioventricular junction
◆ Ventricular: Usually 100 to 150 beats/minute but can be lesser than 100 beats/minute

P WAVE
◆ Absent
◆ Replaced by baseline fibrillatory waves that represent atrial tetanization from rapid atrial depolarizations (see shaded area above)

PR INTERVAL
◆ Indiscernible

QRS COMPLEX
◆ Duration and configuration usually normal

T WAVE
◆ Indiscernible

QT INTERVAL
◆ Not measurable

OTHER
◆ Atrial rhythm may vary between fibrillatory line and flutter waves, called *atrial fibflutter*
◆ May be difficult to differentiate atrial fibrillation from atrial flutter and multifocal atrial tachycardia

---

Alert *Left untreated, atrial fibrillation can lead to cardiovascular collapse, thrombus formation, and systemic arterial or pulmonary embolism. (See* Risk of restoring sinus rhythm.*)*

SIGNS AND SYMPTOMS
The radial pulse rate may be slower than the apical rate because the weaker contractions that occur in atrial fibrillation don't produce a palpable peripheral pulse; only the stronger ones do.

The pulse rhythm will be irregularly irregular, with a normal or abnormal heart rate. Patients with a new onset of atrial fibrillation and a rapid ventricular rate may demonstrate signs and symptoms of decreased cardiac output, including hypotension and light-headedness. Patients with chronic atrial fibrillation may be able to compensate for the decreased cardiac output and may be asymptomatic.

TREATMENT

Treatment of atrial fibrillation aims to reduce the ventricular response rate to less than 100 beats/minute by either administering drugs to control the ventricular response, or by combining electric cardioversion and drug therapy as a way of converting the arrhythmia to normal sinus rhythm. When the onset of atrial fibrillation is acute and the patient can cooperate, vagal maneuvers or carotid sinus massage may slow the ventricular response, but it won't convert the arrhythmia.

If the patient is hemodynamically unstable, synchronized electric cardioversion should be given immediately. Electric cardioversion is most successful if used within the first 48 hours after onset, but is less successful the longer the duration of the arrhythmia.

Alert *Conversion to normal sinus rhythm will cause forceful atrial contractions to resume abruptly. If a thrombus forms in the atria, the resumption of contractions can result in systemic emboli. (See* How synchronized cardioversion works, *page 76.)*

The focus of treatment for hemodynamically stable patients with atrial fibrillation includes controlling the rate, converting the rhythm, and providing anticoagulation if indicated. Specific interventions depend on the patient's cardiac function, whether preexcitation syndromes are involved, and the duration of the arrhythmia.

Drugs to control the ventricular response rate include digoxin and beta-adrenergic blockers and calcium channel blockers. When the rhythm is converted to a normal sinus rhythm, antiarrhythmics such as amiodarone, quinidine, sotalol, and propafenone are used to maintain the rhythm. Some of these drugs prolong the atrial

---

RISK OF RESTORING SINUS RHYTHM

A patient with atrial fibrillation is at increased risk for developing atrial thrombus and subsequent systemic arterial embolism. In atrial fibrillation, neither atrium contracts as a whole. As a result, blood may pool on the atrial wall, and thrombi may form. Thrombus formation places the patient at higher risk for emboli and stroke.

If normal sinus rhythm is restored and the atria contract normally, clots may break away from the atrial wall and travel through the pulmonary or systemic circulation with potentially disastrous results, such as stroke, pulmonary embolism, or coronary arterial occlusion.

---

refractory period, giving the SA node an opportunity to reestablish its role as the heart's pacemaker. Others primarily slow AV node conduction, controlling the ventricular response rate. Nonpharmacologic treatment may include atrial pacing or radiofrequency ablation.

NURSING INTERVENTIONS

- Monitor the patient's heart rate and rhythm. At times, it may be difficult to distinguish atrial fibrillation from MAT and from junctional rhythm. (See *Distinguishing atrial fibrillation from MAT,* page 77, and *Distinguishing atrial fibrillation from junctional rhythm,* page 78.)

Best lead *Lead II is the best choice for monitoring the patient with atrial fibrillation; however, you should be able to identify fibrillation waves and the irregular R-R intervals in most leads.*

- Assess the peripheral and apical pulses. If the patient isn't on a cardiac monitor, be alert for an irregular pulse

HOW SYNCHRONIZED CARDIOVERSION WORKS

A patient experiencing an arrhythmia that leads to reduced cardiac output may be a candidate for synchronized cardioversion. This procedure may be done electively or as an emergency. For instance, it may be used electively in a patient with recurrent atrial fibrillation, or urgently in a patient with ventricular tachycardia and a pulse.

Synchronized cardioversion is similar to defibrillation, also called *unsynchronized cardioversion*. Synchronizing the energy delivered to the patient reduces the risk that the current will strike during the relative refractory period of a cardiac cycle and induce ventricular fibrillation (VF). This vulnerable period occurs early in the T wave.

In synchronized cardioversion, the R wave on the patient's electrocardiogram is synchronized with the cardioverter (defibrillator). Once the firing buttons have been pressed, the cardioverter discharges energy when it senses the next R wave.

Keep in mind that a slight delay occurs between the time the discharge buttons are depressed and the moment the energy is actually discharged. When using handheld paddles, continue to hold the paddles on the patient's chest until the energy is delivered.

Remember to reset the "sync mode" on the defibrillator after each synchronized cardioversion. Resetting this switch is necessary because most defibrillators will automatically reset to an unsynchronized mode.

If VF occurs during the procedure, turn off the sync button and immediately deliver an unsynchronized defibrillation to terminate the arrhythmia. Be aware that synchronized cardioversion carries the risk of lethal arrhythmia when used in patients with digoxin toxicity.

---

and differences in the radial and apical pulse rates.
● Assess for symptoms of decreased cardiac output and heart failure.
● If drug therapy is used, monitor drug levels and observe the patient for evidence of toxicity.
● Tell the patient to report pulse rate changes, syncope or dizziness, chest pain, and signs of heart failure, such as dyspnea and peripheral edema.

Ashman's phenomenon

◆

Ashman's phenomenon refers to the aberrant conduction of premature supraventricular beats to the ventricles. (See *Identifying Ashman's phenomenon,* page 79.) This benign phenomenon is frequently associated with atrial fibrillation but can occur with any arrhythmia that affects the R-R interval.

CAUSES

Ashman's phenomenon is caused by an intermittent bundle-branch block resulting from beat-by-beat loss of conduction. In theory, a conduction aberration occurs when a short cycle follows a long cycle, because the refractory period varies with the length of the cycle. An impulse that ends a short cycle preceded by a long one is more likely to reach refractory tissue.

The normal refractory period for the right bundle branch is slightly longer than the left one, so premature beats frequently reach the right bundle when it's partially or completely refractory. Because of this tendency, the abnormal beat is usually seen as a right bundle-branch block.

DISTINGUISHING ATRIAL FIBRILLATION FROM MAT

To help you decide whether a rhythm is atrial fibrillation, or the similar multifocal atrial tachycardia (MAT), focus on the presence of P waves as well as the atrial and ventricular rhythms. You may find it helpful to look at a longer (more than 6 seconds) rhythm strip.

ATRIAL FIBRILLATION
◆ Carefully look for discernible P waves before each QRS complex.
◆ If you can't clearly identify P waves, and fibrillatory waves (F waves) appear instead of P waves, then the rhythm is probably atrial fibrillation.
◆ Carefully look at the rhythm, focusing on the R-R intervals. Remember that one of the hallmarks of atrial fibrillation is an irregularly irregular rhythm.

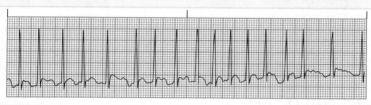

MAT
◆ P waves are present in MAT. Keep in mind, however, that the shape of the P waves will vary, with at least three different P wave shapes visible in a single rhythm strip.
◆ You should be able to see most, if not all, of the various P wave shapes repeat.
◆ Although the atrial and ventricular rhythms are irregular, the irregularity typically isn't as pronounced as in atrial fibrillation.

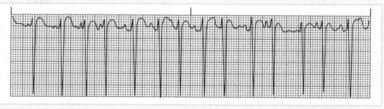

CLINICAL SIGNIFICANCE
The importance of recognizing aberrantly conducted beats is primarily to prevent misdiagnosis and subsequent mistaken treatment of ventricular ectopy.

SIGNS AND SYMPTOMS
No signs and symptoms are found in this phenomenon.

TREATMENT
No treatment is necessary, but treatment may be needed for accompanying arrhythmias.

NURSING INTERVENTIONS
● Monitor heart rate and rhythm.

DISTINGUISHING ATRIAL FIBRILLATION FROM JUNCTIONAL RHYTHM

At times, it can be easy to mistake atrial fibrillation for junctional rhythm. Here's how to tell the two apart.

ATRIAL FIBRILLATION

◆ Examine lead II, which provides a clear view of atrial activity. Look for fibrillatory waves (F waves), which appear as a wavy line. These waves indicate atrial fibrillation.
◆ Chronic atrial fibrillation tends to have fine or small F waves and a controlled ventricular rate (less than 100 beats/minute).

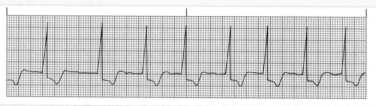

JUNCTIONAL RHYTHM

◆ In lead II, if you can find inverted P waves after or within 0.12 second before the QRS complex (see shaded area below), the rhythm is junctional.
◆ Assess the patient's jugular veins. Look at the A waves, the normally dominant positive waves in the jugular venous waveform. If cannon A waves are seen with each beat, the rhythm is most likely junctional. Cannon A waves are large A waves, indicating that the right atrium is contracting against an increased resistance. Large A waves can occur during arrhythmias whenever the right atrium contracts while the tricuspid valve is closed by right ventricular systole. Regularly occurring cannon A waves may be seen during junctional rhythm, whereas A waves are absent in patients with atrial fibrillation.

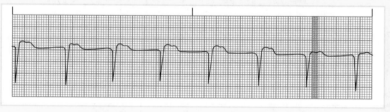

Wandering pacemaker

Wandering pacemaker (also called *wandering atrial pacemaker*) is an atrial arrhythmia caused by the shift in site of impulse formation from the SA node to another area above the ventricles. The origin of the impulse may wander beat to beat from the SA node to ectopic sites in the atria, or to the AV junctional tissue. The P wave and PR interval vary from beat to beat as the pacemaker site changes. (See *Identifying wandering pacemaker,* page 80.)

IDENTIFYING ASHMAN'S PHENOMENON

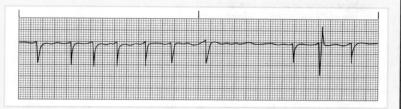

RHYTHM
◆ Atrial: Irregular
◆ Ventricular: Irregular

RATE
◆ Reflects the underlying rhythm

P WAVE
◆ May be visible
◆ Abnormal configuration
◆ Unchanged if present in the underlying rhythm

PR INTERVAL
◆ Commonly changes on the premature beat, if measurable at all

QRS COMPLEX
◆ Altered configuration with right bundle-branch block (RBBB) pattern

T WAVE
◆ Deflection opposite that of QRS complex in most leads because of RBBB

QT INTERVAL
◆ Usually changed because of RBBB

OTHER
◆ No compensatory pause after an aberrant beat
◆ Aberrancy possibly continuing for several beats and typically ends a short cycle preceded by a long cycle

CAUSES
In most cases, wandering pacemaker is caused by increased parasympathetic (vagal) influences on the SA node or AV junction. It can also be caused by chronic pulmonary disease, digoxin toxicity, inflammation of the atrial tissue, and valvular heart disease.

CLINICAL SIGNIFICANCE
The arrhythmia may be normal in young patients and is common in athletes who have slow heart rates. The arrhythmia may be difficult to identify because it's often transient. Although wandering pacemaker is rarely serious, chronic arrhythmias are a sign of heart disease and should be monitored.

SIGNS AND SYMPTOMS
Patients are generally asymptomatic and unaware of the arrhythmia. The pulse rate may be normal or less than 60 beats/minute, and the rhythm may be regular or slightly irregular.

TREATMENT
Usually, no treatment is needed for asymptomatic patients. If the patient is symptomatic, however, his medications should be reviewed and the underlying cause investigated and treated.

IDENTIFYING WANDERING PACEMAKER

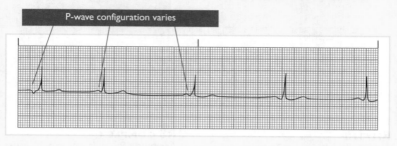

P-wave configuration varies

RHYTHM
◆ Atrial: Varies slightly, with an irregular P-P interval
◆ Ventricular: Varies slightly, with an irregular R-R interval

RATE
◆ Varies, but usually within normal limits or may be less than 60 beats/minute

P WAVE
◆ Altered size and configuration from changing pacemaker site with at least three different P-wave shapes visible
◆ May be absent or inverted or occur after QRS complex if impulse originates in the atrioventricular (AV) junction

PR INTERVAL
◆ Varies from beat to beat as pacemaker site changes

◆ Usually less than 0.20 second
◆ Less than 0.12 second if the impulse originates in the AV junction

QRS COMPLEX
◆ Duration and configuration usually normal because ventricular depolarization is normal

T WAVE
◆ Normal size and configuration

QT INTERVAL
◆ Usually within normal limits

OTHER
◆ May be difficult to differentiate wandering pacemaker from premature atrial contractions

NURSING INTERVENTIONS
● Monitor the patient's heart rate and rhythm. At times it may be difficult to distinguish wandering pacemaker from PACs. (See *Distinguishing wandering pacemaker from PACs.*)
● Watch for signs of hemodynamic instability, such as hypotension and changes in mental status.

Look-alikes

DISTINGUISHING WANDERING PACEMAKER FROM PACs

Because premature atrial contractions (PACs) are commonly encountered, it's possible to mistake a wandering pacemaker for PACs unless the rhythm strip is carefully examined. In such cases, you may find it helpful to look at a longer (more than 6 seconds) rhythm strip.

WANDERING PACEMAKER

◆ Carefully examine the P waves. You must be able to identify at least three different shapes of P waves (see shaded areas below) in wandering pacemaker.
◆ Atrial rhythm varies slightly, with an irregular P-P interval. Ventricular rhythm varies slightly, with an irregular R-R interval. These slight variations in rhythm result from the changing site of impulse formation.

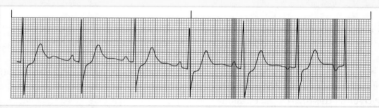

PAC

◆ The PAC occurs earlier than the sinus P wave, with an abnormal configuration when compared with a sinus P wave (see shaded area below). It's possible, but rare, to see multifocal PACs, which originate from multiple ectopic pacemaker sites in the atria. In this setting, the P waves may have different shapes.
◆ With the exception of the irregular atrial and ventricular rhythms as a result of the PAC, the underlying rhythm is usually regular.

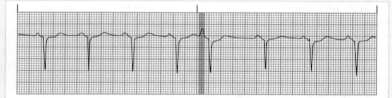

6

JUNCTIONAL ARRHYTHMIAS

Junctional arrhythmias originate in the atrioventricular (AV) junction—the area in and around the AV node and the bundle of His. The specialized pacemaker cells in the AV junction take over as the heart's pacemaker if the sinoatrial (SA) node fails to function properly, or if the electrical impulses originating in the SA node are blocked. These junctional pacemaker cells have an inherent firing rate of 40 to 60 beats/minute.

In normal impulse conduction, the AV node slows transmission of the impulse from the atria to the ventricles, which allows the ventricles to fill as much as possible before they contract. However, these impulses don't always follow the normal conduction pathway. (See *Conduction in Wolff-Parkinson-White syndrome.*)

Because of the location of the AV junction within the conduction pathway, electrical impulses that originate in this area cause abnormal depolarization of the heart. The impulse is conducted in a retrograde (backward) fashion to depolarize the atria, and antegrade (forward) to depolarize the ventricles.

Depolarization of the atria can precede depolarization of the ventricles, or the ventricles can be depolarized before the atria. Depolarization can also occur simultaneously in the atria and ventricles. (See *Locating the P wave,* page 84.) Retrograde depolarization of the atria results in inverted P waves in leads II, III, and aV_F, leads in which you would normally see upright P waves appear.

Keep in mind that arrhythmias causing inverted P waves on an electrocardiogram (ECG) may originate in the atria or AV junction. Atrial arrhythmias are sometimes mistaken for junctional arrhythmias because impulses are generated so low in the atria that they cause retrograde depolarization and inverted P waves. Looking at the PR interval will help you determine whether an arrhythmia is atrial or junctional.

An arrhythmia with an inverted P wave before the QRS complex and with a normal PR interval (0.12 to 0.20 second) originates in the atria. An arrhythmia with a PR interval less than 0.12 second originates in the AV junction.

CONDUCTION IN WOLFF-PARKINSON-WHITE SYNDROME

Electrical impulses in the heart don't always follow normal conduction pathways. In pre-excitation syndromes, electrical impulses enter the ventricles from the atria through an accessory pathway that bypasses the atrioventricular junction. Wolff-Parkinson-White (WPW) syndrome is a common type of preexcitation syndrome.

WPW syndrome commonly occurs in young children and in adults ages 20 to 35. The syndrome causes the PR interval to shorten and the QRS complex to lengthen as a result of a delta wave. Delta waves, which in WPW occur just before normal ventricular depolarization, are produced as a result of the premature depolarization or preexcitation of a portion of the ventricles.

WPW is clinically significant because the accessory pathway—in this case, Kent's bundle—may result in paroxysmal tachyarrhythmias by reentry and rapid conduction mechanisms.

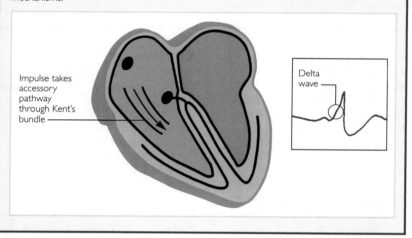

Impulse takes accessory pathway through Kent's bundle

Delta wave

Premature junctional contractions

A premature junctional contraction (PJC) is a junctional beat that occurs before a normal sinus beat and causes an irregular rhythm. These ectopic beats commonly occur as a result of enhanced automaticity in the junctional tissue or bundle of His. As with all impulses generated in the AV junction, the atria are depolarized in a retrograde fashion, causing an inverted P wave. The ventricles are depolarized normally. (See *Identifying premature junctional contractions,* page 85.)

CAUSES
PJCs may be caused by:
- alcohol
- amphetamines
- chronic pulmonary disease
- coronary artery disease
- digoxin toxicity
- electrolyte imbalances

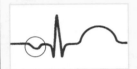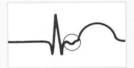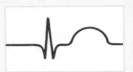
- excessive caffeine
- heart failure
- hyperthyroidism
- inflammatory changes in AV junction
- myocardial ischemia
- pericarditis
- stress
- valvular heart disease.

CLINICAL SIGNIFICANCE

Infrequent PJCs are generally considered harmless.

Alert *Frequent PJCs indicate junctional irritability and can precipitate a more serious arrhythmia, such as junctional tachycardia. In patients taking digoxin, PJCs are a common early sign of toxicity.*

SIGNS AND SYMPTOMS

The patient is usually asymptomatic. He may complain of palpitations or a feeling of "skipped heart beats." You may be able to palpate an irregular pulse when PJCs occur. If PJCs are frequent enough, the patient may experience hypotension from a transient decrease in cardiac output.

TREATMENT

PJCs usually don't require treatment unless the patient is symptomatic. In those cases, the underlying cause should be treated. For example, in digoxin toxicity, you should discontinue digoxin and monitor drug levels in the blood. If ectopic beats occur because of caffeine, the patient should decrease or eliminate caffeine.

NURSING INTERVENTIONS

- Monitor heart rate and rhythm.
- Monitor the patient for hemodynamic instability.

Junctional rhythm

A junctional rhythm, also referred to as a *junctional escape rhythm,* is an arrhythmia that originates in the AV junction. In this arrhythmia, the AV junction takes over as a secondary, or "escape" pacemaker. This usually occurs only when a higher pacemaker site in the atria, typically the SA node, fails as the heart's dominant pacemaker.

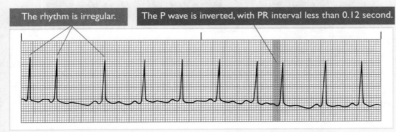

IDENTIFYING PREMATURE JUNCTIONAL CONTRACTIONS

The rhythm is irregular.

The P wave is inverted, with PR interval less than 0.12 second.

RHYTHM
- Atrial: Irregular during premature junctional contractions (PJCs)
- Ventricular: Irregular during PJCs
- Underlying rhythm possibly regular

RATE
- Atrial: Reflects underlying rhythm
- Ventricular: Reflects underlying rhythm

P WAVE
- Usually inverted (leads II, III, and aV$_F$) (see shaded area above)
- May occur before, during, or after QRS complex, depending on initial direction of depolarization
- May be hidden in QRS complex

PR INTERVAL
- Shortened (less than 0.12 second) if P wave precedes QRS complex
- Not measurable if no P wave precedes QRS complex

QRS COMPLEX
- Usually normal configuration and duration because ventricles usually depolarize normally

T WAVE
- Usually normal configuration

QT INTERVAL
- Usually within normal limits

OTHER
- Commonly accompanied by a compensatory pause reflecting retrograde atrial conduction

Remember that the AV junction can take over as the heart's dominant pacemaker if the firing rate of the higher pacemaker sites falls below the AV junction intrinsic firing rate, if the pacemaker fails to generate an impulse, or if the conduction of the impulses is blocked. Because junctional escape beats prevent ventricular standstill, they should never be suppressed.

In a junctional rhythm, as in all junctional arrhythmias, the atria are depolarized by means of retrograde conduction. The P waves are inverted, and impulse conduction through the ventricles is normal. The normal intrinsic firing rate for cells in the AV junction is 40 to 60 beats/minute. (See *Identifying junctional rhythm,* page 86.)

Junctional escape beats may occur in healthy children during sleep or in healthy athletic adults. In these situations, no treatment is necessary.

CAUSES
A junctional escape rhythm can be caused by any condition that disturbs normal SA node function or impulse

IDENTIFYING JUNCTIONAL RHYTHM

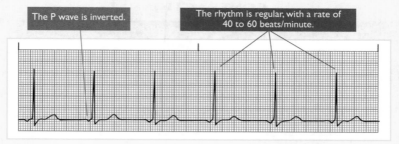

The P wave is inverted.

The rhythm is regular, with a rate of 40 to 60 beats/minute.

RHYTHM
- Atrial: Regular
- Ventricular: Regular

RATE
- Atrial: 40 to 60 beats/minute
- Ventricular: 40 to 60 beats/minute

P WAVE
- Usually inverted (leads II, III, and aV_F)
- May occur before, during, or after QRS complex
- May be hidden in QRS complex

PR INTERVAL
- Shortened (less than 0.12 second) if P wave precedes QRS complex

- Not measurable if no P wave precedes QRS complex

QRS COMPLEX
- Duration: Usually within normal limits
- Configuration: Usually normal

T WAVE
- Configuration: Usually normal

QT INTERVAL
- Usually within normal limits

OTHER
- Important to differentiate junctional rhythm from idioventricular rhythm (a life-threatening arrhythmia)

conduction. Causes of the arrhythmia include:
- cardiomyopathy
- electrolyte imbalances
- heart failure
- hypoxia
- increased parasympathetic (vagal) tone
- myocarditis
- SA node ischemia
- sick sinus syndrome
- valvular heart disease.

Drugs, such as digoxin, calcium channel blockers, and beta-adrenergic blockers, can also cause a junctional escape rhythm.

CLINICAL SIGNIFICANCE

The clinical significance of junctional rhythm depends on how well the patient tolerates a decreased heart rate (40 to 60 beats/minute) and associated decrease in cardiac output. In addition, depolarization of the atria either after or simultaneously with ventricular depolarization results in loss of atrial kick. Remember that junctional escape rhythms protect the heart from potentially life-threatening ventricular escape rhythms.

SIGNS AND SYMPTOMS

A patient with a junctional rhythm will have a slow, regular pulse rate of

40 to 60 beats/minute. The patient may be asymptomatic.

🔵 **Alert** *Pulse rates less than 60 beats/minute may lead to inadequate cardiac output, causing hypotension, syncope, or blurred vision.*

TREATMENT

Treatment for a junctional rhythm involves identification and correction of the underlying cause, whenever possible. (For specific treatments, see the Bradycardia algorithm, page 262.) Atropine may be used to increase the heart rate while waiting for a temporary or permanent pacemaker to be inserted.

NURSING INTERVENTIONS

● Monitor heart rate and rhythm. Junctional rhythm can sometimes be difficult to distinguish from atrial fibrillation with third-degree block. (See *Distinguishing atrial fibrillation with third-degree AV block from junctional rhythm,* page 88.)
● Monitor the patient's digoxin and electrolyte levels in the blood.
● Watch for signs of decreased cardiac output, such as hypotension, syncope, and blurred vision.

Accelerated junctional rhythm

An accelerated junctional rhythm is an arrhythmia that originates in the AV junction and is usually caused by enhanced automaticity of the AV junctional tissue. It's called accelerated because it occurs at a rate of 60 to 100 beats/minute, exceeding the inherent junctional escape rate of 40 to 60 beats/minute.

Because the rate is less than 100 beats/minute, the arrhythmia isn't classified as junctional tachycardia. The atria are depolarized by means of retrograde conduction, and the ventricles are depolarized normally. (See *Identifying accelerated junctional rhythm,* page 89.)

CAUSES

Digoxin toxicity is a common cause of accelerated junctional rhythm. Other causes include:
● cardiac surgery
● electrolyte disturbances
● heart failure
● inferior- or posterior-wall myocardial infarction
● myocarditis
● rheumatic heart disease
● valvular heart disease.

CLINICAL SIGNIFICANCE

Patients experiencing accelerated junctional rhythm are generally asymptomatic because the rate corresponds to the normal inherent firing rate of the SA node (60 to 100 beats/minute). However, symptoms of decreased cardiac output, including hypotension and syncope, can occur if atrial depolarization occurs after or simultaneously with ventricular depolarization, which causes the subsequent loss of atrial kick.

SIGNS AND SYMPTOMS

The pulse rate will be normal with a regular rhythm. The patient may be asymptomatic because accelerated junctional rhythm has the same rate as sinus rhythm. However, if cardiac output is decreased, the patient may exhibit symptoms, such as hypotension, changes in mental status, and weak peripheral pulses.

Distinguishing atrial fibrillation with third-degree AV block from junctional rhythm

Although third-degree atrioventricular (AV) block occurs infrequently, it can happen in association with atrial fibrillation. The resulting ventricular rhythm will be regular. If the block occurs at the level of the AV node, a junctional escape pacemaker usually initiates ventricular depolarization. This event results in a normally shaped, narrow QRS complex and a ventricular rate of 40 to 60 beats/minute.

Differentiating the cause of the arrhythmias is vital because even though the escape rhythm is a junctional rhythm, patient management of the conditions may differ.

Atrial fibrillation with third-degree AV block
◆ On lead II, which provides a clear view of atrial activity, search for fibrillatory waves (f waves) indicating atrial fibrillation.
◆ Assess the patient's jugular veins; A waves will be absent with atrial fibrillation.

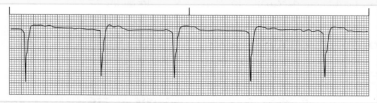

Junctional rhythm
◆ Inverted P waves either after or within 0.12 second before the QRS complex on lead II indicate junctional rhythm.
◆ Assess the patient's jugular veins; large a waves, called *cannon a waves*, occur with junctional rhythm.

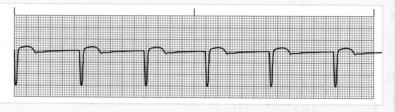

Treatment
Accelerated junctional rhythm can be treated by identifying and correcting the underlying cause.

Nursing interventions
● Monitor heart rate and rhythm.
● Watch for evidence of decreased cardiac output and hemodynamic instability.

● Monitor serum digoxin and electrolyte levels.

Junctional tachycardia

In junctional tachycardia, three or more premature PJCs occur in a row.

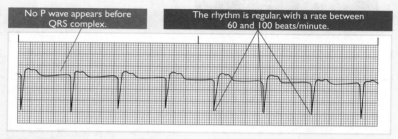

IDENTIFYING ACCELERATED JUNCTIONAL RHYTHM

No P wave appears before QRS complex.

The rhythm is regular, with a rate between 60 and 100 beats/minute.

RHYTHM
◆ Atrial: Regular
◆ Ventricular: Regular

RATE
◆ Atrial: 60 to 100 beats/minute
◆ Ventricular: 60 to 100 beats/minute

P WAVE
◆ If present, inverted in leads II, III, and aV$_F$
◆ May occur before, during, or after QRS complex
◆ May be hidden in QRS complex

PR INTERVAL
◆ Shortened (less than 0.12 second) if P wave precedes QRS complex

◆ Not measurable if no P wave precedes QRS complex

QRS COMPLEX
◆ Duration: Usually within normal limits
◆ Configuration: Usually normal

T WAVE
◆ Usually within normal limits

QT INTERVAL
◆ Usually within normal limits

OTHER
◆ Important to differentiate accelerated junctional rhythm from accelerated idioventricular rhythm (a possibly life-threatening arrhythmia)

This supraventricular tachycardia generally occurs as a result of enhanced automaticity of the AV junction, which causes the AV junction to override the SA node as the dominant pacemaker.

In junctional tachycardia, the atria are depolarized by retrograde conduction. Conduction through the ventricles is normal. The rate is usually 100 to 200 beats/minute. (See *Identifying junctional tachycardia,* page 90.)

CAUSES
Digoxin toxicity is the most common cause of junctional tachycardia. In such cases, the arrhythmia can be aggravated by hypokalemia. Other causes include:
● electrolyte imbalances
● heart failure
● inferior- or posterior-wall infarction or ischemia
● inflammation of the AV junction following heart surgery
● valvular heart disease.

CLINICAL SIGNIFICANCE
The clinical significance of junctional tachycardia depends on the rate and underlying cause. At higher ventricular rates, junctional tachycardia may re-

IDENTIFYING JUNCTIONAL TACHYCARDIA

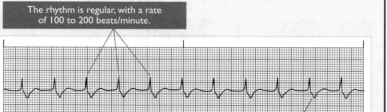

The rhythm is regular, with a rate of 100 to 200 beats/minute.

The P wave occurs after QRS complex.

RHYTHM

◆ Atrial: Usually regular, but may be difficult to determine if P wave is hidden in QRS complex or preceding T wave
◆ Ventricular: Usually regular

RATE

◆ Atrial: Greater than 100 beats/minute (usually 100 to 200 beats/minute), but may be difficult to determine if P wave is hidden in QRS complex
◆ Ventricular: Greater than 100 beats/minute (usually 100 to 200 beats/minute)

P WAVE

◆ Usually inverted in leads II, III, and aV$_F$
◆ May occur before, during, or after QRS complex
◆ May be hidden in QRS complex

PR INTERVAL

◆ Shortened (less than 0.12 second) if P wave precedes QRS complex
◆ Not measurable if no P wave precedes QRS complex

QRS COMPLEX

◆ Duration: Within normal limits
◆ Configuration: Usually normal

T WAVE

◆ Configuration: Usually normal
◆ May be abnormal if P wave is hidden in T wave
◆ May be indiscernible because of fast rate

QT INTERVAL

◆ Usually within normal limits

OTHER

◆ May have gradual onset

duce cardiac output by decreasing ventricular filling time. A loss of atrial kick also occurs with atrial depolarization that follows or occurs simultaneously with ventricular depolarization.

SIGNS AND SYMPTOMS

The patient's pulse rate will be greater than 100 beats/minute and have a regular rhythm.

Alert *Patients with a rapid heart rate may experience signs and symptoms of decreased cardiac output and hemodynamic instability, including hypotension.*

TREATMENT

The underlying cause should be identified and treated. If the cause is digoxin toxicity, digoxin should be stopped; however, digoxin may be used if it isn't the cause of the tachycardia. Patients with recurrent junctional tachycardia may be treated with ablation therapy, followed by permanent pacemaker insertion.

If symptomatic with paroxysmal onset of junctional tachycardia, vagal maneuvers and drugs such as adenosine may slow the heart rate. If the patient has normal heart function, beta-adrenergic blockers, calcium channel blockers, or amiodarone may be administered.

NURSING INTERVENTIONS
- Monitor heart rate and rhythm.
- Watch for signs of decreased cardiac output.
- Watch for evidence of digoxin toxicity and monitor serum digoxin levels.

7

VENTRICULAR ARRHYTHMIAS

Ventricular arrhythmias originate in the ventricles below the bifurcation of the bundle of His. These arrhythmias occur when electrical impulses depolarize the myocardium using a different pathway from normal impulse conduction.

Ventricular arrhythmias appear on an electrocardiogram (ECG) in characteristic ways. The QRS complex in most of these arrhythmias is wider than normal because of the prolonged conduction time through, and abnormal depolarization of, the ventricles. The deflections of the T wave and the QRS complex are in opposite directions because ventricular repolarization, as well as ventricular depolarization, is abnormal. The P wave in many ventricular arrhythmias is absent because atrial depolarization doesn't occur. If a P wave is present, it originates in the sinus node, causing it to be dissociated from the ventricular rhythm.

When electrical impulses come from the ventricles instead of the atria, atrial kick is lost and cardiac output can decrease by as much as 30%. As a result, patients with ventricular arrhythmias may show signs and symptoms of decreased cardiac output, in-cluding hypotension, angina, syncope, and respiratory distress.

Although ventricular arrhythmias may be benign, they also may be serious because the ventricles are ultimately responsible for cardiac output. Rapid recognition and treatment of ventricular arrhythmias increases the chances of successful return to normal rhythm.

Premature ventricular contractions

Premature ventricular contractions (PVCs) are ectopic beats that originate in the ventricles and occur earlier than expected. PVCs may occur in healthy people without being clinically significant.

However, when PVCs occur in patients with underlying heart disease, they may indicate development of lethal ventricular arrhythmias, including ventricular tachycardia (VT) and ventricular fibrillation (VF).

PVCs may occur singly, in pairs (couplets), or in clusters. PVCs may also appear in patterns, such as bi-

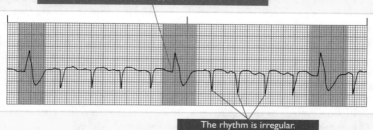

IDENTIFYING PVCs

Premature QRS complex appears wide and bizarre.

The rhythm is irregular.

RHYTHM
- Atrial: Irregular during premature ventricular contractions (PVCs)
- Ventricular: Irregular during PVCs
- Underlying rhythm may be regular

RATE
- Atrial: Reflects underlying rhythm
- Ventricular: Reflects underlying rhythm

P WAVE
- Usually absent in ectopic beat
- May appear after QRS complex with retrograde conduction to atria
- Usually normal if present in underlying rhythm

PR INTERVAL
- Not measurable except in underlying rhythm

QRS COMPLEX
- Occurs earlier than expected
- Duration: Greater than 0.12 second
- Configuration: Wide and bizarre with PVC (see shaded areas)
- Usually normal in underlying rhythm

T WAVE
- Opposite direction to QRS complex
- May trigger more serious rhythm disturbances when PVC occurs on the downslope of the preceding normal T wave (R-on-T phenomenon)

QT INTERVAL
- Not usually measured except in underlying rhythm

OTHER
- PVC may be followed by full or occasionally an incomplete compensatory pause
- Full compensatory pause existing if the P-P interval encompassing the PVC has twice the duration of a normal sinus beat's P-P interval.
- Incomplete compensatory pause existing if the P-P interval encompassing the PVC is less than twice the duration of a normal sinus beat's P-P interval
- Interpolated PVC: Occurs between two normally conducted QRS complexes without great disturbance to underlying rhythm
- Full compensatory pause absent with interpolated PVCs
- May be difficult to distinguish PVCs from aberrant ventricular conduction

geminy or trigeminy. (See *Identifying PVCs*.) In many cases, PVCs are followed by a compensatory pause because the timing from the sinoatrial (SA) node isn't interrupted. PVCs may be uniform, arising from a single ectopic ventricular pacemaker site, or multiform, with QRS complexes different in size, shape, and direction, indicating a different pattern of ventricular depolarization.

PVCs also may be described as unifocal or multifocal. Unifocal PVCs originate from the same ventricular ectopic pacemaker site, whereas multifocal PVCs originate from different ectopic pacemaker sites in the ventricles.

Causes

PVCs may be caused by enhanced or abnormal automaticity in the ventricular conduction system or muscle tissue. The irritable focus is caused by a disruption of the normal electrolyte shifts during cellular depolarization and repolarization. Possible causes of PVCs include:
- alcohol
- caffeine
- drug intoxication, particularly with cocaine, amphetamines, and tricyclic antidepressants
- electrolyte imbalances, such as hypokalemia, hyperkalemia, hypomagnesemia, or hypocalcemia
- enlargement or hypertrophy of the ventricular chambers
- hypoxia
- increased sympathetic stimulation
- irritation of the ventricles by pacemaker electrodes or a pulmonary artery catheter
- metabolic acidosis
- myocardial ischemia and infarction
- myocarditis
- proarrhythmic effects of some antiarrhythmics
- sympathomimetic drugs, such as epinephrine and isoproterenol
- tobacco.

Clinical significance

PVCs are significant for two reasons. First, they can lead to more serious arrhythmias, such as VT or VF. The risk of developing a more serious arrhythmia increases in patients with ischemic or damaged hearts or with significant electrolyte imbalance.

PVCs also decrease cardiac output, especially if ectopic beats are frequent or repetitive. The decrease in cardiac output with a PVC stems from reduced ventricular diastolic filling time and the loss of atrial kick for that beat. The clinical impact of PVCs hinges on the body's ability to maintain adequate perfusion and the duration of the abnormal rhythm.

To help determine the seriousness of PVCs, ask yourself these questions:
- How often do they occur? In patients with chronic PVCs, an increase in frequency or a change in the pattern of PVCs from the baseline rhythm may signal a more serious condition.
- What's the pattern of PVCs? If the ECG shows a dangerous pattern—such as paired PVCs, PVCs with more than one focus, a bigeminal rhythm, or R-on-T phenomenon (when a PVC strikes on the down slope of the preceding normal T wave)—the patient may require immediate treatment. (See *Patterns of potentially dangerous PVCs*.)
- Are they really PVCs? Make sure the complex is a PVC and not another, less dangerous arrhythmia. PVCs may be mistaken for ventricular escape beats or normal impulses with aberrant ventricular conduction. Ventricular escape beats serve as a safety mechanism to protect the heart from ventricular standstill. Some supraventricular impulses may follow an abnormal conduction pathway, causing an abnormal appearance to the QRS complex. In any event, never delay treatment if the patient is unstable.

Patterns of
Potentially Dangerous PVCs

Some premature ventricular contractions (PVCs) are more dangerous than others. Here are examples of patterns of potentially dangerous PVCs.

Paired PVCs

Two PVCs in a row, called *paired PVCs* or a *ventricular couplet* (see shaded areas below), can produce ventricular tachycardia (VT). That's because the second contraction usually meets refractory tissue. A burst, or *salvo*, of three or more PVCs in a row is considered a run of VT.

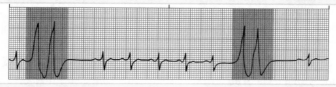

Multiform PVCs

Multiform PVCs, which look different from one another, arise from different sites or from the same site with abnormal conduction (see shaded areas below). Multiform PVCs may indicate severe heart disease or digoxin toxicity.

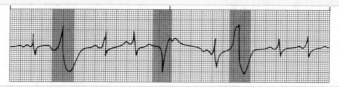

Bigeminy and Trigeminy

PVCs that occur every other beat (*bigeminy*) or every third beat (*trigeminy*) may indicate increased ventricular irritability, which can result in VT or ventricular fibrillation (see shaded areas below). The rhythm strip shown below illustrates ventricular bigeminy.

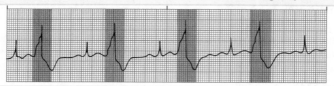

R-on-T phenomenon

In R-on-T phenomenon, a PVC occurs so early that it falls on the T wave of the preceding beat (see shaded area below). Because the cells haven't fully repolarized, VT or ventricular fibrillation can result.

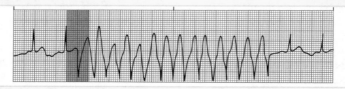

SIGNS AND SYMPTOMS

A patient with PVCs usually has a pulse rate within the normal range of 60 to 100 beats/minute. When a PVC occurs, the pulse rhythm will be momentarily irregular.

With PVCs, the patient will have a weaker pulse wave after the premature beat and a longer-than normal pause between pulse waves. At times, you may not be able to palpate a pulse after the PVC. If the carotid pulse is visible, however, you may see a weaker arterial wave after the premature beat. When auscultating for heart sounds, you'll hear an abnormally early heart sound with each PVC.

A patient with PVCs may be asymptomatic. However, patients with frequent PVCs may complain of palpitations. The patient also may exhibit signs and symptoms of decreased cardiac output, including hypotension and syncope.

TREATMENT

If the PVCs are infrequent and the patient has normal heart function and is asymptomatic, the arrhythmia probably won't require treatment. If symptoms of a dangerous form of PVCs occur, the type of treatment given will depend on the cause of the problem.

If PVCs have a purely cardiac origin, drugs to suppress ventricular irritability such as procainamide, amiodarone, and lidocaine are typically used. When PVCs have a noncardiac origin, treatment is aimed at correcting the cause. For example, drug therapy may be adjusted or the patient's acidosis or electrolyte imbalance corrected.

NURSING INTERVENTIONS

● Monitor ECG rhythm. Sometimes it's difficult to distinguish PVCs from aberrant ventricular conduction. (See *Distinguishing PVCs from ventricular aberrancy*.)

✳ **Best lead** *Leads V_1, V_6, MCL_1, and MCL_6 are the best choices for identifying PVCs.*

● Promptly assess patients with recently developed PVCs, especially if they have underlying heart disease or complex medical problems.

● Observe closely for the development of more frequent PVCs or more dangerous PVC patterns and notify the practitioner of changes.

● Teach family members how to contact the emergency medical system, and encourage them to learn cardiopulmonary resuscitation (CPR).

Idioventricular rhythm

Idioventricular rhythm (also called *ventricular escape rhythm*) originates in an escape pacemaker site in the ventricles. The inherent firing rate of this ectopic pacemaker is usually 30 to 40 beats/minute. The rhythm acts as a safety mechanism by preventing ventricular standstill, or asystole—the absence of electrical activity in the ventricles. When fewer than three QRS complexes arising from the escape pacemaker occur, they're called ventricular escape beats or complexes. (See *Identifying idioventricular rhythm,* page 98.)

When the rate of an ectopic pacemaker site in the ventricles is less than 100 beats/minute but is greater than the inherent ventricular escape rate of 30 to 40 beats/minute, it's called accelerated idioventricular rhythm (AIVR). (See *Identifying accelerated idioventricular rhythm,* page 99.) The rate of AIVR

DISTINGUISHING PVCs FROM VENTRICULAR ABERRANCY

One of the most challenging look-alikes—premature ventricular contractions (PVCs) versus ventricular aberrancy—can sometimes be distinguished with complete confidence only in the electrophysiology laboratory. Ventricular aberrancy, or aberrant ventricular conduction, occurs when an electrical impulse originating in the sinoatrial node, atria, or atrioventricular junction is temporarily conducted abnormally through the bundle branches.

The abnormal conduction results in a bundle-branch block and usually stems from the arrival of electrical impulses at the bundle branches before the branches have been sufficiently repolarized.

To distinguish between PVCs and ventricular aberrancy, examine the deflection of the QRS complex in lead V_1. Determine whether the QRS complex is primarily positive or negative. Based on this information, follow these clues to guide your analysis.

MOSTLY POSITIVE QRS

◆ Right bundle-branch aberrancy will have a triphasic rSR′ configuration in V_1 and a triphasic qRS configuration in V_6.

◆ If there are two positive peaks in V_1 and the left peak is taller, the beat is probably a PVC.
◆ PVCs will be monophasic or biphasic in V_1, and biphasic in V_6, with a deep S wave.

COMPARING PVC WITH RIGHT BUNDLE-BRANCH ABERRANCY

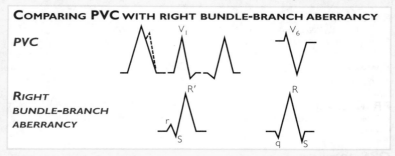

MOSTLY NEGATIVE QRS

◆ Left bundle-branch aberrancy will have a narrow R wave with a quick downstroke in leads V_1 and V_2, and no Q wave in V_6.
◆ PVCs will have a wide R wave (> 0.03 second) and a notched or slurred S-wave downstroke in leads V_1 and V_2, with a duration of > 0.06 second from the onset of the R wave to the deepest point of the S wave in V_1 and V_2, and a Q wave in V_6.
◆ P waves commonly precede aberrancies. P waves don't generally precede PVCs.
◆ Aberrancies usually have a QRS duration of 0.12 to 0.14 second. PVCs are more likely to have a QRS duration of 0.16 second or more.

COMPARING PVC WITH LEFT BUNDLE-BRANCH ABERRANCY

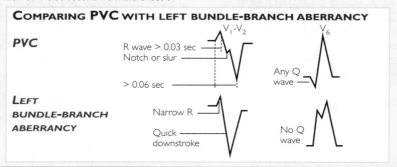

IDENTIFYING IDIOVENTRICULAR RHYTHM

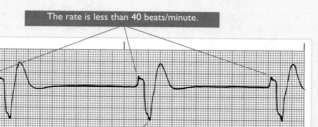

The rate is less than 40 beats/minute.

The QRS complex is wide and bizarre.

RHYTHM
◆ Atrial: Usually can't be determined
◆ Ventricular: Usually regular

RATE
◆ Atrial: Usually can't be determined
◆ Ventricular: 20 to 40 beats/minute

P WAVE
◆ Usually absent

PR INTERVAL
◆ Not measurable because of absent P wave

QRS COMPLEX
◆ Duration: Greater than 0.12 second because of abnormal ventricular depolarization
◆ Configuration: Wide and bizarre

T WAVE
◆ Abnormal
◆ Usually deflects in opposite direction from QRS complex

QT INTERVAL
◆ Usually prolonged

OTHER
◆ Commonly occurs with third-degree atrioventricular block
◆ If any P waves present, not associated with QRS complex

---

isn't fast enough to be considered VT. The rhythm is usually related to enhanced automaticity of the ventricular tissue. AIVR and idioventricular rhythm share the same ECG characteristics, differing only in heart rate. Because the rate of AIVR is similar to a normal heart rate, the patient is usually asymptomatic.

CAUSES

Idioventricular rhythms occur when all of the heart's higher pacemakers fail to function or when supraventricular impulses can't reach the ventricles because of a block in the conduction system. Idioventricular rhythms may accompany third-degree heart block. Possible causes of the rhythm include:
● digoxin toxicity, beta-adrenergic blockers, calcium antagonists, and tricyclic antidepressants

Life-threatening

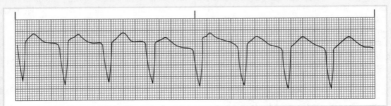

IDENTIFYING ACCELERATED IDIOVENTRICULAR RHYTHM

RHYTHM
◆ Atrial: Can't be determined
◆ Ventricular: Usually regular

RATE
◆ Atrial: Usually can't be determined
◆ Ventricular: 40 to 100 beats/minute

P WAVE
◆ Usually absent

PR INTERVAL
◆ Not measurable

QRS COMPLEX
◆ Duration: Greater than 0.12 second
◆ Configuration: Wide and bizarre

T WAVE
◆ Abnormal
◆ Usually deflects in opposite direction from QRS complex

QT INTERVAL
◆ Usually prolonged

OTHER
◆ If any P waves present, not associated with QRS complex

- metabolic imbalances
- myocardial infarction (MI)
- myocardial ischemia
- pacemaker failure.

CLINICAL SIGNIFICANCE
Idioventricular rhythm may be transient or continuous. Transient ventricular escape rhythm is usually related to increased parasympathetic effect on the higher pacemaker sites and isn't generally clinically significant.

Although idioventricular rhythms act to protect the heart from ventricular standstill, a continuous idioventricular rhythm presents a clinically serious situation.

 Alert *The slow ventricular rate of this arrhythmia and the associated*

loss of atrial kick markedly reduce cardiac output. If not rapidly identified and appropriately managed, idioventricular arrhythmias can cause death.

SIGNS AND SYMPTOMS
The patient with continuous idioventricular rhythm is generally symptomatic because of the marked reduction in cardiac output that occurs with the arrhythmia. Blood pressure may be difficult or impossible to auscultate or palpate. The patient may experience dizziness, light-headedness, syncope, or loss of consciousness.

TRANSCUTANEOUS PACEMAKER

Transcutaneous pacing, also referred to as *external pacing* or *noninvasive pacing*, involves the delivery of electrical impulses through externally applied cutaneous electrodes. The electrical impulses are conducted through an intact chest wall using skin electrodes placed either in anterior-posterior or sternal-apex positions. (An anterior-posterior placement is shown here.)

Transcutaneous pacing is the initial pacing method of choice in emergency situations because it's the least invasive technique and it can be instituted quickly.

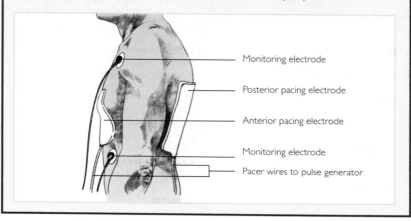

- Monitoring electrode
- Posterior pacing electrode
- Anterior pacing electrode
- Monitoring electrode
- Pacer wires to pulse generator

TREATMENT

Treatment should be initiated immediately to increase the patient's heart rate, improve cardiac output, and establish a normal rhythm. Atropine may be administered to increase the heart rate.

If atropine isn't effective or if the patient develops hypotension or other signs of clinical instability, a pacemaker may be needed to reestablish a heart rate that provides enough cardiac output to perfuse organs properly. A transcutaneous pacemaker may be used in an emergency until a temporary or transvenous pacemaker can be inserted. (See *Transcutaneous pacemaker.*)

Alert *Remember, the goal of treatment doesn't include suppressing the idioventricular rhythm, because it acts as a safety mechanism to protect the heart from* *ventricular standstill. Idioventricular rhythm should never be treated with lidocaine or other antiarrhythmics that would suppress the escape beats.*

NURSING INTERVENTIONS

- Monitor ECG continually. Sometimes it may be difficult to distinguish AIVR from accelerated junctional rhythm. (See *Distinguishing AIVR from accelerated junctional rhythm.*)
- Closely assess the patient until treatment restores hemodynamic stability.
- Keep atropine and pacemaker equipment available at the patient's bedside.
- Enforce bed rest until an effective heart rate has been maintained and the patient is clinically stable.
- Tell the patient and family members about the serious nature of this

DISTINGUISHING AIVR FROM ACCELERATED JUNCTIONAL RHYTHM

Accelerated idioventricular rhythm (AIVR) and accelerated junctional rhythm appear similar, but they have different causes. To distinguish between the two, closely examine the duration of the QRS complex and then look for P waves.

AIVR

◆ The QRS duration will be greater than 0.12 second.
◆ The QRS will have a wide and bizarre configuration.
◆ P waves are usually absent.
◆ The ventricular rate is generally between 40 and 100 beats/minute.

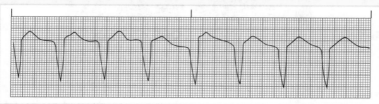

ACCELERATED JUNCTIONAL RHYTHM

◆ The QRS duration and configuration are usually normal.
◆ Inverted P waves generally occur before or after the QRS complex. However, remember that the P waves may also appear absent when hidden within the QRS complex.
◆ The ventricular rate is typically between 60 and 100 beats/minute.

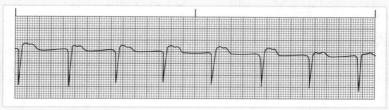

arrhythmia and the treatment it requires.

● If the patient needs a permanent pacemaker, teach the patient and family how it works, how to recognize problems, when to contact the practitioner, and how pacemaker function will be monitored.

Ventricular tachycardia

VT (also called *V-tach*) occurs when three or more PVCs strike in a row and the ventricular rate is greater than 100 beats/minute. This life-threatening arrhythmia usually precedes VF and sudden cardiac death, especially in patients who aren't in a health care facility.

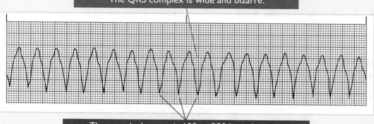

IDENTIFYING VT

The QRS complex is wide and bizarre.

The ventricular rate is 100 to 250 beats/minute.

RHYTHM
◆ Atrial: Can't be determined
◆ Ventricular: Usually regular but may be slightly irregular

RATE
◆ Atrial: Can't be determined
◆ Ventricular: Usually rapid (100 to 250 beats/minute)

P WAVE
◆ Usually absent
◆ If present, not associated with QRS complex

PR INTERVAL
◆ Not measurable

QRS COMPLEX
◆ Duration: Greater than 0.12 second
◆ Configuration: Usually bizarre, with increased amplitude
◆ Uniform in monomorphic ventricular tachycardia (VT)
◆ Constantly changes shape in polymorphic VT

T WAVE
◆ Not discernible

QT INTERVAL
◆ Not measurable

OTHER
◆ Ventricular flutter (VF): A variation of VT
◆ Torsades de pointes: A variation of polymorphic VT that's sometimes difficult to distinguish from VF

VT is an extremely unstable rhythm and may be sustained or nonsustained. When it occurs in short, paroxysmal bursts lasting less than 30 seconds and causing few or no symptoms, it's called nonsustained. When the rhythm is sustained, however, it requires immediate treatment to prevent death, even in patients initially able to maintain adequate cardiac output. (See *Identifying VT.*)

CAUSES

This arrhythmia is usually caused by increased myocardial irritability, which may be triggered by enhanced automaticity, reentry within the Purkinje system, or by PVCs occurring during the downstroke of the preceding T wave.

Other causes of VT include:
● cardiomyopathy
● coronary artery disease (CAD)

- drug intoxication from procainamide, quinidine, or cocaine
- electrolyte imbalances such as hypokalemia
- heart failure
- MI
- myocardial ischemia
- proarrhythmic effects of some antiarrhythmics
- valvular heart disease.

CLINICAL SIGNIFICANCE

VT is significant because of its unpredictability and potential for causing death. A patient may be hemodynamically stable, with a normal pulse and blood pressure; clinically unstable, with hypotension and poor peripheral pulses; or unconscious, without respirations or pulse.

Because of the reduced ventricular filling time and the drop in cardiac output that occurs with this arrhythmia, the patient's condition can quickly deteriorate to ventricular fibrillation and complete cardiovascular collapse.

SIGNS AND SYMPTOMS

Although some patients at first have only minor symptoms, they still require rapid intervention to prevent cardiovascular collapse. Most patients with VT have weak or absent pulses. Low cardiac output will cause hypotension and a decreased level of consciousness, quickly leading to unresponsiveness if left untreated. VT may prompt angina, heart failure, or a substantial decrease in organ perfusion.

TREATMENT

Treatment depends on the patient's clinical status. Is the patient conscious? Does the patient have spontaneous respirations? Is a palpable carotid pulse present?

Alert *Patients with pulseless VT are treated the same as those with ventricular fibrillation and require immediate defibrillation and CPR. Treatment for patients with a detectable pulse depends on whether they're stable or unstable.*

Unstable patients generally have ventricular rates greater than 150 beats/minute and have serious signs and symptoms related to the tachycardia, which may include hypotension, shortness of breath, chest pain, or altered consciousness. These patients are usually treated with immediate synchronized cardioversion.

A clinically stable patient with VT and no signs of heart failure is treated differently. Treatment for these patients is determined by whether the rhythm is regular or irregular. If the rhythm is regular (monomorphic), the patient is treated with amiodarone and possible synchronized cardioversion. If the rate is irregular (polymorphic), look at the length of the QT interval when the rhythm is in sinus rhythm. If the QT interval is long, the polymorphic rhythm is most likely torsades de pointes. (See *Identifying torsades de pointes,* page 104, and *Distinguishing ventricular flutter from torsades de pointes,* page 105.)

The treatment for polymorphic VT is to stop medications that may cause a long QT, correct electrolyte imbalances, and administer an antiarrhythmic, such as magnesium or amiodarone. If at any point the patient becomes clinically unstable, immediate synchronized cardioversion is the best treatment.

Patients with VT or VF not from a transient or reversible cause may need

Life-threatening

IDENTIFYING TORSADES DE POINTES

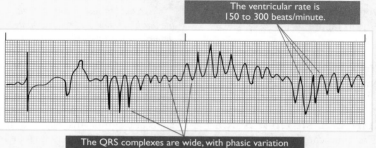

The ventricular rate is 150 to 300 beats/minute.

The QRS complexes are wide, with phasic variation that seems to twist around the baseline.

RHYTHM
◆ Atrial: Can't be determined
◆ Ventricular: May be regular or irregular

RATE
◆ Atrial: Can't be determined
◆ Ventricular: 150 to 300 beats/minute

P WAVE
◆ Not identifiable

PR INTERVAL
◆ Not measurable

QRS COMPLEX
◆ Usually wide

◆ Usually a phasic variation of electrical polarity, with complexes that point downward for several beats and then upward for several beats

T WAVE
◆ Not discernible

QT INTERVAL
◆ Not measurable

OTHER
◆ May be paroxysmal, starting and stopping suddenly

an implanted cardioverter-defibrillator (ICD). This device is a permanent solution to recurrent episodes of VT.

A 12-lead ECG and all other available clinical information are critical for establishing a specific diagnosis in a stable patient with wide QRS complex tachycardia of unknown type but regular rate. If a definitive diagnosis of supraventricular tachycardia or VT can't be established, amiodarone (to control the rate) and elective synchronized cardioversion are used.

NURSING INTERVENTIONS
● Determine if the patient is conscious and has spontaneous respirations and palpable carotid pulse.
● Initiate CPR and advanced life support measures as necessary.
● Monitor heart rate and rhythm. The rhythm may rapidly progress to ventricular fibrillation. Sometimes distinguishing VT from supraventricular tachycardia can be very challenging, especially in the setting of aberrant ventricular conduction. (See *Distinguishing VT from SVT,* pages 106 and 107.)

Look-alikes

DISTINGUISHING VENTRICULAR FLUTTER FROM TORSADES DE POINTES

Although rarely recognized, ventricular flutter is caused by the rapid, regular, repetitive beating of the ventricles. It's produced by a single ventricular focus firing at a rapid rate of 250 to 350 beats/minute. The hallmark of this arrhythmia is its smooth sine-wave appearance.

Torsades de pointes is a variant form of ventricular tachycardia, with a rapid ventricular rate that varies between 150 and 300 beats/minute. It's characterized by QRS complexes that gradually change back and forth, with the amplitude of each successive complex gradually increasing and decreasing. This results in an overall outline of the rhythm commonly described as spindle-shaped.

The illustrations shown here highlight key differences in the two arrhythmias.

VENTRICULAR FLUTTER
◆ Smooth, sine-wave appearance

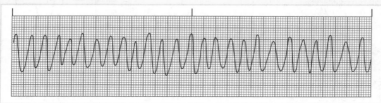

TORSADES DE POINTES
◆ Spindle-shaped appearance

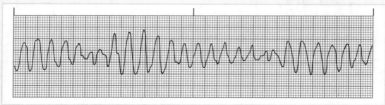

Best lead *Leads V_1 and V_6, or the modified chest leads MCL_1 and MCL_6, are the best leads for monitoring the patient with VT.*

● Teach the patient and his family about the serious nature of this arrhythmia and the need for prompt treatment.

● If your stable patient is undergoing electrical cardioversion, inform him

that he'll be given a sedative and possibly an analgesic before the procedure.

Alert *If a patient will be discharged with an ICD or a prescription for long-term antiarrhythmics, make sure that family members know how to use the emergency medical system and how to perform CPR.*

(Text continues on page 108.)

Look-alikes

DISTINGUISHING VT FROM SVT

Differentiating ventricular tachycardia (VT) from supraventricular tachycardia (SVT) with aberrancy is difficult. Careful assessment of a 12-lead electrocardiogram or rhythm strip can help you differentiate the arrhythmia with 90% accuracy.

Begin by looking at the deflection—negative or positive, and then use the following illustrations to guide your assessment. If the QRS complex is wide and mostly negative in deflection in V_1 or MCL_1, use these clues:

VT
◆ If the QRS complex has an R wave ≥ 0.04 second, a slurred S (shown below, shaded), or a notched S (shown below at right) on the downstroke, suspect VT.

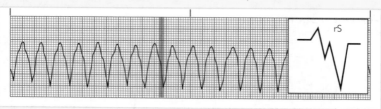

SVT
◆ If the QRS complex has an R wave ≤ 0.04 second and a swift, straight S on the downstroke (shown below, shaded, and below right), suspect SVT with aberrancy.

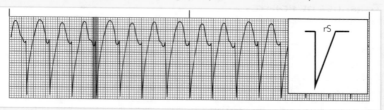

If the QRS complex is wide and mostly positive in deflection in V_1 or MCL_1, use these clues:

VT
◆ If the QRS complex is biphasic, suspect VT.

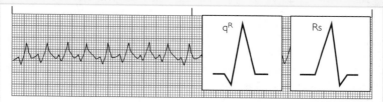

SVT

◆ If the beat is triphasic, similar to a right bundle-branch block, suspect SVT with aberrancy.

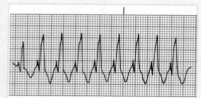
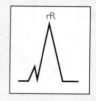
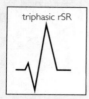

Other clues you can use if the QRS complex is wide and mostly positive in deflection in lead V_1 or MCL_1 include the following:

If the QRS complex is tall and shaped like rabbit ears, with the left peak taller than the right, suspect VT.

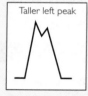

If the QRS complex is monophasic, suspect VT.

If you still have trouble differentiating the rhythm, look at V_6 or MCL_6.

If the S wave is larger than the R wave, suspect VT.

If any Q wave is present, suspect VT.

OTHER GENERAL CRITERIA CAN ALSO HELP YOU DIFFERENTIATE VT FROM SVT WITH ABERRANCY.

◆ A QRS complex > 0.14 second suggests VT.
◆ A regular, wide, complex rhythm suggests VT.
◆ An irregular, wide, complex rhythm suggests SVT with aberrancy.
◆ Concordant V leads (the QRS complex either mainly positive or mainly negative in all V leads) suggest VT.
◆ Atrioventricular dissociation suggests VT.

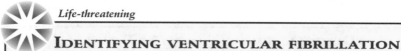

IDENTIFYING VENTRICULAR FIBRILLATION

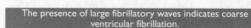

The presence of large fibrillatory waves indicates coarse ventricular fibrillation.

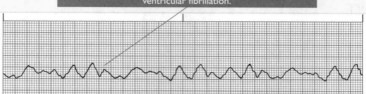

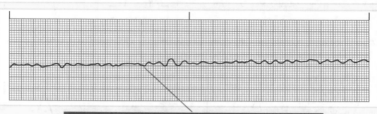

The presence of small fibrillatory waves indicates fine ventricular fibrillation.

RHYTHM
◆ Atrial: Not measurable
◆ Ventricular: No pattern or regularity, just fibrillatory waves

RATE
◆ Atrial: Not measurable
◆ Ventricular: Not measurable

P WAVE
◆ Not visible

PR INTERVAL
◆ Not measurable

QRS COMPLEX
◆ Not measurable

T WAVE
◆ Not measurable

QT INTERVAL
◆ Not measurable

OTHER
◆ Electrical defibrillation: more successful with coarse fibrillatory waves than with fine waves, which indicate more advanced hypoxemia and acidosis

Ventricular fibrillation

Ventricular fibrillation (VF), also called *V-fib,* is characterized by a chaotic, disorganized pattern of electrical activity. The pattern arises from electrical impulses coming from multiple ectopic pacemakers in the ventricles.

The arrhythmia produces no effective ventricular mechanical activity or contractions and no effective cardiac output. Untreated VF is the most common cause of sudden cardiac death in people outside of a health care facility. (See *Identifying ventricular fibrillation.*)

CAUSES

Causes of VF include:

- acid-base imbalance
- CAD
- drug toxicity, including digoxin, quinidine, and procainamide
- electric shock
- electrolyte imbalances, such as hypokalemia, hyperkalemia, and hypercalcemia
- MI
- myocardial ischemia
- severe hypothermia
- severe hypoxia
- underlying heart disease
- untreated VT.

CLINICAL SIGNIFICANCE

With VF, the ventricular muscle quivers, replace effective muscular contraction with completely ineffective contraction. Cardiac output falls to zero and, if allowed to continue, leads to ventricular standstill and death.

SIGNS AND SYMPTOMS

The patient in VF is in full cardiac arrest, unresponsive, and without a detectable blood pressure or central pulses. Whenever you see an ECG pattern resembling VF, check the patient immediately and initiate definitive treatment.

TREATMENT

Immediate defibrillation and CPR are the most effective treatments for VF. CPR must be performed until the defibrillator arrives to preserve oxygen supply to the brain and other vital organs, and after the first attempt at defibrillation. After a cycle of CPR, a second defibrillation is attempted. Defibrillators vary by facility and may deliver monophasic or biphasic current. (See *Monophasic and biphasic defibrillators*, page 110.)

Drugs, such as epinephrine and vasopressin, may be used for persistent VF if the first two attempts at defibrillation are unsuccessful. Antiarrhythmics, such as amiodarone, lidocaine, and magnesium, may also be considered. (For specific treatment, see Pulseless arrest algorithm, page 260.)

In defibrillation, two electrode pads or paddles are applied to the chest wall. Current is then directed through the pads into the patient's chest and heart. The current causes the myocardium to completely depolarize, which, in turn, encourages the SA node to resume normal control of the heart's electrical activity.

For anterolateral placement, one electrode pad or paddle is placed to the right of the upper sternum, and one is placed over the fifth or sixth intercostal space at the left anterior axillary line. For anteroposterior placement, one electrode pad or paddle is placed directly over the heart at the precordium, to the left of the sternal border, and one is placed under the patient's body beneath the heart and just below the left scapula. During cardiac surgery, internal paddles are placed directly on the myocardium.

Automated external defibrillators (AEDs) are increasingly being used, especially in the out-of-hospital setting, to provide early defibrillation. After a patient is confirmed to be unresponsive, breathless, and pulseless, the AED power is turned on and the electrode pads and cables attached. The AED can analyze the patient's cardiac rhythm and provide the caregiver with step-by-step instructions on how to proceed. These defibrillators can be used by people without

Monophasic and biphasic defibrillators

Monophasic defibrillators

Monophasic defibrillators deliver a single current of electricity that travels in one direction between the two pads or paddles on the patient's chest. To be effective, a large amount of electrical current is required for monophasic defibrillation.

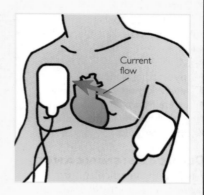

Current flow

Biphasic defibrillators

Biphasic defibrillators have the same pad or paddle placement as monophasic defibrillators. The difference is that during biphasic defibrillation, the electric current discharged from the pads or paddles travels in a positive direction for a specified duration and then reverses and flows in a negative direction for the remainder of the electrical discharge. Some of the advantages of the biphasic system are described below.

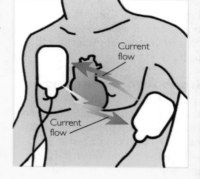

Current flow

Current flow

Energy efficient

The biphasic defibrillator delivers two currents of electricity and lowers the defibrillation threshold of the heart muscle, making it possible to successfully defibrillate ventricular fibrillation (VF) with smaller amounts of energy.

Adjustable

The biphasic defibrillator can adjust for differences in impedance or resistance of the current through the chest. This reduces the number of shocks needed to terminate VF.

Less myocardial damage

Because the biphasic defibrillator requires lower energy levels and fewer shocks, damage to the myocardial muscle is reduced. Biphasic defibrillators used at the clinically appropriate energy level may be used for defibrillation and, in the synchronized mode, for synchronized cardioversion.

medical experience as long as they're trained in the proper use of the device. (See *Automated external defibrillators.*)

Nursing interventions

- When faced with a rhythm that appears to be VF, first assess the pa-

AUTOMATED EXTERNAL DEFIBRILLATORS

Automated external defibrillators (AEDs) vary by manufacturer, but the basic components of each device are similar. This illustration shows a typical AED and how to place electrodes properly.

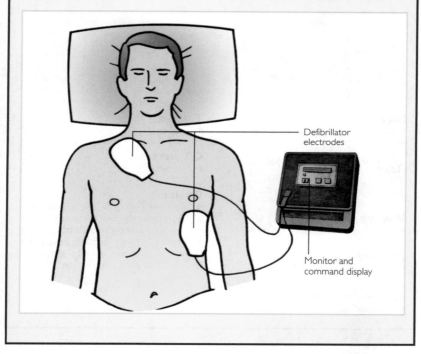

Defibrillator electrodes

Monitor and command display

tient. Other events can mimic VF on an ECG strip, including interference from an electric razor, shivering, or seizure activity.

● Start CPR.

● Teach the patient and family how to use the emergency medical system following discharge from the facility. Family members may need instruction in CPR.

● Teach the patient and family about long-term therapies that help prevent recurrent episodes of VF, including antiarrhythmic drug therapy and ICDs.

Asystole

Ventricular asystole, also called *asystole* and *ventricular standstill,* is the absence of discernible electrical activity in the ventricles. Although some electrical activity may be evident in the atria, these impulses aren't conducted to the ventricles. (See *Identifying asystole,* page 112.)

Asystole usually results from a prolonged period of cardiac arrest without effective resuscitation.

IDENTIFYING ASYSTOLE

The absence of electrical activity in the ventricles results in a nearly flat line.

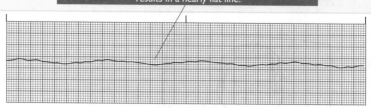

RHYTHM
♦ Atrial: Usually indiscernible
♦ Ventricular: Not present

RATE
♦ Atrial: Usually indiscernible
♦ Ventricular: Not present

P WAVE
♦ Usually indiscernible

PR INTERVAL
♦ Not measurable

QRS COMPLEX
♦ Absent or occasional escape beats

T WAVE
♦ Absent

QT INTERVAL
♦ Not measurable

OTHER
♦ Looks like a nearly flat line on a rhythm strip except during chest compressions with cardiopulmonary resuscitation
♦ If the patient has pacemaker, pacer spikes may show on the strip, but no P wave or QRS complex occurs in response

Alert *It's important to distinguish asystole from fine VF, which is managed differently. Therefore, asystole must be confirmed in more than one ECG lead.*

CAUSES
Possible reversible causes of asystole include:
● cardiac tamponade
● drug overdose
● hypothermia
● hypovolemia
● hypoxia
● massive pulmonary embolism
● MI (coronary thrombosis)
● severe electrolyte disturbances, especially hyperkalemia and hypokalemia
● severe, uncorrected acid-base disturbances, especially metabolic acidosis
● tension pneumothorax.

CLINICAL SIGNIFICANCE
Without ventricular electrical activity, ventricular contractions can't occur. As a result, cardiac output drops to zero and vital organs are no longer perfused. Asystole has been called the arrhythmia of death and is typically considered to be a confirmation of

PULSELESS ELECTRICAL ACTIVITY

Pulseless electrical activity (PEA), also referred to as *electromechanical dissociation (EMD)* or *non-perfusing rhythm*, defines a group of arrhythmias characterized by the presence of some type of electrical activity, but with no detectable pulse. Although organized electrical depolarization occurs, no synchronous shortening of the myocardial fibers occurs. As a result, no mechanical activity or contractions take place. Included in the PEA category are the aforementioned EMD as well as pseudo-EMD, idioventricular rhythms, and ventricular escape rhythms.

CAUSES

The most common causes of PEA include hypovolemia, hypoxia, acidosis, tension pneumothorax, cardiac tamponade, massive pulmonary embolism, hypothermia, hyperkalemia and hypokalemia, massive acute myocardial infarction, severe trauma, electrocution, and overdoses of drugs such as tricyclic antidepressants.

TREATMENT

Rapid identification and treatment of underlying reversible causes is critical for treating PEA. For example, hypovolemia is treated with volume expansion. Tension pneumothorax is treated with needle decompression.

Institute cardiopulmonary resuscitation immediately and administer I.V. epinephrine or vasopressin. Atropine may be given if the PEA rate is slow.

---

death, rather than an arrhythmia to be treated.

The patient with asystole is completely unresponsive, without spontaneous respirations or pulse (cardiopulmonary arrest). Without immediate start of CPR and rapid identification and treatment of the underlying cause, the condition quickly becomes irreversible.

SIGNS AND SYMPTOMS

The patient will be unresponsive and have no spontaneous respirations, discernible pulse, or blood pressure.

TREATMENT

Immediate treatment for asystole includes effective CPR and supplemental oxygen. Resuscitation should be attempted unless evidence exists that these efforts shouldn't be initiated, such as when a do-not-resuscitate

order is in effect. (See Pulseless arrest algorithm, page 260.)

Priority must also be given to searching for and treating identified potentially reversible causes. Early CPR is vital, and I.V., intraosseous epinephrine, or a one-time dose of vasopressin and atropine is given.

Pulseless electrical activity also can lead to asystole. (See *Pulseless electrical activity.*)

With persistent asystole despite appropriate management, consideration should be given to terminating resuscitation.

NURSING INTERVENTIONS
● Verify the presence of asystole by checking more than one ECG lead.
● Verify lack of do-not-resuscitate order.
● Start CPR and advanced life support measures.

8

ATRIOVENTRICULAR BLOCKS

Atrioventricular (AV) heart block refers to a permanent or transient interruption or delay in the conduction of electrical impulses between the atria and the ventricles. The block can occur at the AV node, the bundle of His, or the bundle branches. When the site of block is the bundle of His or the bundle branches, the block is referred to as *infranodal* AV block. AV block can be partial (first or second degree) or complete (third degree).

Causes and classifications of AV blocks

The heart's electrical impulses normally originate in the sinoatrial (SA) node, so when those impulses are blocked at the AV node, atrial rates are often normal (60 to 100 beats/minute). The clinical significance of the block depends on the number of impulses that are completely blocked, and the resulting ventricular rate. A slow ventricular rate can decrease cardiac output and cause symptoms such as light-headedness, hypotension, and confusion.

CAUSES OF AV BLOCK

A variety of factors may lead to AV block, including underlying heart conditions, use of certain drugs, congenital anomalies, and conditions that disrupt the cardiac conduction system.

Typical causes of AV block include:
● cardiomyopathies, myocarditis, and cardiac tumors
● congenital anomalies, such as congenital ventricular septal defects that involve cardiac structures and affect the conduction system (Anomalies of the conduction system, such as an AV node that doesn't conduct impulses, also can occur in the absence of structural defects.)
● excessive blood levels of, or an exaggerated response to, a drug (This response can cause AV block or increase the likelihood that a block will develop. The drugs may increase the refractory period of a portion of the conduction system. Although many antiarrhythmics can have this effect, the drugs more commonly known to cause or exacerbate AV blocks include digoxin, beta-adrenergic blockers and calcium channel blockers, and amiodarone.)
● increased vagal tone caused by pain, carotid sinus massage, or a

hypersensitive carotid sinus (These can slow the sinus node and lead to an AV block.)

- lesions (including calcified and fibrotic lesions) along the conduction pathway
- myocardial infarction (MI), in which cellular necrosis or death occurs (If the necrotic cells are part of the conduction system, they may no longer conduct impulses and a permanent AV block occurs.)
- myocardial ischemia, which impairs cellular function so that cells repolarize more slowly or incompletely (The injured cells, in turn, may conduct impulses slowly or inconsistently. Relief of the ischemia may restore normal function to the AV node.).

In elderly patients, AV block may be caused by fibrosis of the conduction system. Other causes include the use of digoxin and the presence of aortic valve calcification.

AV block also can be caused by inadvertent damage to the heart's conduction system during cardiac surgery. Damage is most likely to occur during surgery involving the mitral or tricuspid valve or in the closure of a ventricular septal defect. If the injury involves tissues adjacent to the surgical site and the conduction system isn't physically disrupted, the block may be only temporary. If a portion of the conduction system itself is severed, permanent block results.

Similar disruption of the conduction system can occur from a procedure called radiofrequency ablation. In this invasive procedure, a transvenous catheter is used to locate the area in the heart that participates in initiating or perpetuating certain tachyarrhythmias. Radiofrequency energy is then delivered to the myocardium through this catheter to produce a small area of necrosis at that spot. The damaged tissue can no longer cause or participate in the tachyarrhythmia. If the energy is delivered close to the AV node, bundle of His, or bundle branches, however, AV block can result.

CLASSIFICATION OF AV BLOCK

AV blocks are classified according to the site of block and the severity of the conduction abnormality. The sites of AV block include the AV node, bundle of His, and bundle branches.

Severity of AV block is classified in degrees:
- first-degree AV block
- second-degree AV block
- type I (Wenckebach or Mobitz I)
- type II (Mobitz II)
- third-degree (complete) AV block.

The classification system for AV blocks aids in the determination of the patient's treatment and prognosis.

First-degree AV block

First-degree AV block occurs when there's a delay in the conduction of electrical impulses from the atria to the ventricles. This delay usually occurs at the level of the AV node, but it also may be infranodal. First-degree AV block is characterized by a PR interval greater than 0.20 second. This interval usually remains constant beat to beat. Electrical impulses are conducted through the normal conduction pathway. However, conduction of these impulses takes longer than normal.

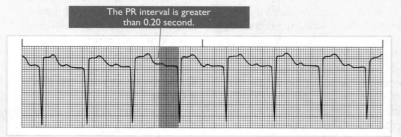

IDENTIFYING FIRST-DEGREE AV BLOCK

The PR interval is greater than 0.20 second.

RHYTHM
◆ Regular

RATE
◆ Within normal limits
◆ Atrial the same as ventricular

P WAVE
◆ Normal size
◆ Normal configuration
◆ Each followed by a QRS complex

PR INTERVAL
◆ Prolonged
◆ Greater than 0.20 second (see shaded area above)
◆ Constant

QRS COMPLEX
◆ Within normal limits (0.08 second) if conduction delay occurs in atrioventricular (AV) node
◆ If greater than 0.12 second, conduction delay may be in His-Purkinje system

T WAVE
◆ Normal size
◆ Normal configuration
◆ May be abnormal if QRS complex is prolonged

QT INTERVAL
◆ Within normal limits

OTHER
◆ None

CAUSES

First-degree AV block may result from:
● degenerative changes in the heart associated with aging
● drugs, such as beta-adrenergic blockers, calcium channel blockers, and digoxin
● myocardial infarction
● myocardial ischemia
● myocarditis.

CLINICAL SIGNIFICANCE

First-degree AV block may cause no symptoms in a healthy person. The arrhythmia may be transient, espe-cially if it occurs secondary to drugs or ischemia early in the course of an MI. The presence of first-degree block, the least dangerous type of AV block, in-dicates a delay in the conduction of electrical impulses through the normal conduction pathway. In general, a rhythm strip with this block looks like a normal sinus rhythm, except that the PR interval is longer than normal.

Alert Because first-degree AV block can progress to a more severe type of AV block, the patient's cardiac rhythm should be monitored for changes. (See Identifying first-degree AV block.)

SIGNS AND SYMPTOMS

The patient's pulse rate will usually be normal and the rhythm will be regular. Most patients with first-degree AV block are asymptomatic because cardiac output isn't significantly affected. If the PR interval is extremely long, a longer interval between S_1 and S_2 may be noted on cardiac auscultation.

TREATMENT

Treatment generally focuses on identification and correction of the underlying cause. For example, if a drug is causing the AV block, the dosage may be reduced or the drug discontinued. Close monitoring can help detect progression of first-degree AV block to a more serious form of block.

NURSING INTERVENTIONS

● Observe the electrocardiogram (ECG) for progression of the block to a more severe form.
● Administer digoxin, calcium channel blockers, and beta-adrenergic blockers cautiously.

Second-degree AV block, type I

Also called *Wenckebach* or *Mobitz I block,* type I second-degree AV block occurs when each successive impulse from the SA node is delayed slightly longer than the previous impulse. (See *Identifying type I second-degree AV block,* page 118.) This pattern of progressive prolongation of the PR interval continues until an impulse fails to be conducted to the ventricles.

Usually only a single impulse is blocked from reaching the ventricles, and following this nonconducted P wave or dropped beat, the pattern is repeated. This repetitive sequence of two or more consecutive beats followed by a dropped beat results in "group beating." Type I second-degree AV block generally occurs at the level of the AV node.

CAUSES

Type I second-degree AV block frequently results from increased parasympathetic tone or the effects of certain drugs. Coronary artery disease, inferior-wall MI, and rheumatic fever may increase parasympathetic tone and result in the arrhythmia. It may also be caused by cardiac medications, such as beta-adrenergic blockers, calcium channel blockers, and digoxin.

CLINICAL SIGNIFICANCE

Type I second-degree AV block may occur normally in an otherwise healthy person. It also may occur in patients with a high vagal tone, in athletes at rest, or in elderly patients. Almost always transient, this type of block usually resolves when the underlying condition is corrected. Although an asymptomatic patient with this block has a good prognosis, the block may progress to a more serious form, especially if it occurs early in an MI.

SIGNS AND SYMPTOMS

Usually asymptomatic, a patient with type I second-degree AV block may show signs and symptoms of decreased cardiac output, such as light-headedness or hypotension. Symptoms may be especially pronounced if the ventricular rate is slow.

TREATMENT

Treatment is rarely needed because the patient is generally asymptomatic. For a patient with serious signs and

IDENTIFYING TYPE I SECOND-DEGREE AV BLOCK

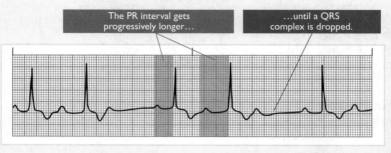

The PR interval gets progressively longer...

...until a QRS complex is dropped.

RHYTHM
◆ Atrial: Regular
◆ Ventricular: Irregular

RATE
◆ Atrial rate exceeds ventricular rate because of nonconducted beats
◆ Both rates usually within normal limits

P WAVE
◆ Normal size
◆ Normal configuration
◆ Each followed by a QRS complex except blocked P wave

PR INTERVAL
◆ Progressively longer (see shaded areas) with each cycle until a P wave appears without a QRS complex
◆ Commonly described as "long, longer, dropped"
◆ Slight variation in delay from cycle to cycle

◆ After the nonconducted beat, shorter than the interval preceding it

QRS COMPLEX
◆ Usually within normal limits
◆ Periodically absent

T WAVE
◆ Normal size
◆ Normal configuration
◆ Deflection may be opposite that of the QRS complex

QT INTERVAL
◆ Usually within normal limits

OTHER
◆ Wenckebach pattern of grouped beats (footprints of Wenckebach)
◆ PR interval gets progressively longer and R-R interval shortens until a P wave appears without a QRS complex; cycle then repeats

---

symptoms related to a low heart rate, atropine may be used to improve AV node conduction. A transcutaneous pacemaker may be required for a symptomatic patient until the arrhythmia resolves. (See Bradycardia algorithm, page 262.)

NURSING INTERVENTIONS
● Check the ECG frequently to see if a more severe type of AV block develops.
● Monitor the tolerance for the rhythm.
● Observe for signs and symptoms of decreased cardiac output.
● Provide patient teaching about a temporary pacemaker, if indicated.

Second-degree AV block, type II

Type II second-degree AV block (also known as *Mobitz II block*) is less common than type I, but more serious. It occurs when impulses from the SA node occasionally fail to conduct to the ventricles. This form of second-degree AV block occurs below the level of the AV node, either at the bundle of His, or more commonly at the bundle branches.

One of the hallmarks of this type of block is that, unlike type I second-degree AV block, the PR interval doesn't lengthen before a dropped beat. (See *Identifying type II second-degree AV block,* page 120.) In addition, more than one nonconducted beat can occur in succession.

CAUSES

Unlike type I second-degree AV block, type II second-degree AV block rarely results from increased parasympathetic tone or drug effects. Type II second-degree AV block is commonly caused by an anterior-wall MI, degenerative changes in the conduction system, or severe coronary artery disease.

CLINICAL SIGNIFICANCE

Unlike type I second-degree AV block, type II second-degree AV block almost always occurs below the AV node and is usually associated with organic heart disease. As a result, this type of block usually is characterized by a poorer prognosis and a greater probability that complete heart block may develop.

In type II second-degree AV block, the ventricular rate tends to be slower than in type I. In addition, cardiac output tends to be lower and symptoms are more likely to appear, particularly if the sinus rhythm is slow and the ratio of conducted beats to dropped beats is low, such as 2:1.

SIGNS AND SYMPTOMS

Most patients who experience occasional dropped beats remain asymptomatic as long as cardiac output is maintained. As the number of dropped beats increases, the patient may experience signs and symptoms of decreased cardiac output, including fatigue, dyspnea, chest pain, lightheadedness, and syncope. On assessment, you may note hypotension and a slow pulse, with a regular or irregular rhythm.

TREATMENT

If the patient doesn't experience serious signs and symptoms related to the low heart rate, the patient may be prepared for transvenous pacemaker insertion. Alternatively, the patient may be continuously monitored, with a transcutaneous pacemaker readily available.

If the patient is experiencing serious signs and symptoms caused by bradycardia, treatment goals include improving cardiac output by increasing the heart rate. Intravenous atropine, transcutaneous pacing, I.V. dopamine, or I.V. epinephrine may be used to increase cardiac output. (See Bradycardia algorithm, page 262.)

Because this form of second-degree AV block occurs below the level of the AV node — either at the bundle of His or, more commonly, at the bundle branches — transcutaneous pacing should be initiated quickly, when indicated. For this reason, type II second-degree AV block also may require placement of a permanent

IDENTIFYING TYPE II SECOND-DEGREE AV BLOCK

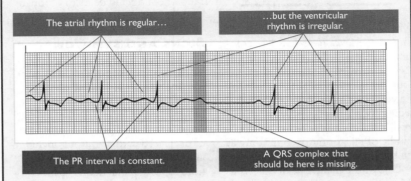

The atrial rhythm is regular...

...but the ventricular rhythm is irregular.

The PR interval is constant.

A QRS complex that should be here is missing.

RHYTHM
◆ Atrial: Regular
◆ Ventricular: Irregular
◆ Pauses correspond to dropped beat
◆ Irregular when block is intermittent or conduction ratio is variable
◆ Regular when conduction ratio is constant, such as 2:1 or 3:1

RATE
◆ Atrial exceeds ventricular
◆ Both may be within normal limits

P WAVE
◆ Normal size
◆ Normal configuration
◆ Some not followed by a QRS complex

PR INTERVAL
◆ Usually within normal limits, but may be prolonged
◆ Constant for conducted beats

QRS COMPLEX
◆ Within normal limits or narrow if block occurs at bundle of His
◆ Widened and similar to bundle-branch block if block occurs at bundle branches
◆ Periodically absent

T WAVE
◆ Normal size
◆ Normal configuration

QT INTERVAL
◆ Within normal limits

OTHER
◆ PR and R-R intervals don't vary before a dropped beat, so no warning occurs
◆ R-R interval that contains nonconducted P wave equals two normal R-R intervals
◆ Must be a complete block in one bundle branch and intermittent interruption in conduction in the other bundle for a dropped beat to occur

---

pacemaker. A temporary pacemaker may be used until a permanent pacemaker can be inserted.

NURSING INTERVENTIONS
● Observe cardiac rhythm for progression to a more severe block. It may be difficult to distinguish

nonconducted PACs from type II second-degree AV block. (See *Distinguishing nonconducted PACs from type II second-degree AV block*.)
● Assess the patient's tolerance of the rhythm and the need for interventions to improve cardiac output and relieve symptoms.

Look-alikes

DISTINGUISHING NONCONDUCTED PACs FROM TYPE II SECOND-DEGREE AV BLOCK

An isolated P wave that doesn't conduct through to the ventricle (P wave without a QRS complex following it; see shaded areas below) may occur with a nonconducted premature atrial contraction (PAC) or may indicate type II second-degree atrioventricular (AV) block. Mistakenly identifying AV block as nonconducted PACs may have serious consequences. Nonconducted PACs are generally benign but type II second-degree AV block can be life-threatening.

NONCONDUCTED PAC
If the P-P interval (including the extra P wave) isn't constant, it's a nonconducted PAC.

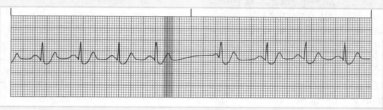

TYPE II SECOND-DEGREE AV BLOCK
If the P-P interval is constant (including the extra P wave), it's type II second-degree AV block.

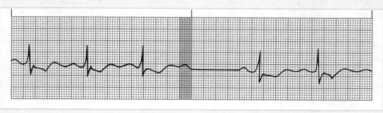

● Keep the patient on bed rest, if indicated, to reduce myocardial oxygen demands.
● Make sure that the patient has a patent I.V. line.
● Administer oxygen therapy, as ordered.
● Keep transcutaneous pacemaker at the bedside, as ordered.
● Teach the patient and family about the use of pacemakers if the patient requires one.

Third-degree AV block

Also called *complete heart block* or *AV dissociation,* third-degree AV block-indicates the complete absence of impulse conduction between the atria and ventricles. In complete heart block, the atrial rate is generally equal to or faster than the ventricular rate.

Third-degree AV block may occur at the level of the AV node, the bundle of His, or the bundle branches. The patient's treatment and prognosis will vary depending on the anatomic level of the block.

When third-degree AV block occurs at the level of the AV node, ventricular depolarization is typically initiated by a junctional escape pacemaker. This pacemaker is usually stable with a rate of 40 to 60 beats/minute. (See *Identifying third-degree AV block*.) The sequence of ventricular depolarization is usually normal because the block is located above the bifurcation of the bundle of His, which results in a normal-appearing QRS complex.

On the other hand, when third-degree AV block occurs at the infranodal level, a block involving the right and left bundle branches is most commonly the cause. In this case, extensive disease exists in the infranodal conduction system, and the only available escape mechanism is located distal to the site of block in the ventricle. This unstable, ventricular escape pacemaker has a slow intrinsic rate of less than 40 beats/minute. Because these depolarizations originate in the ventricle, the QRS complex will have a wide and unusual appearance.

CAUSES

Third-degree AV block occurring at the anatomic level of the AV node can be caused by increased parasympathetic tone associated with inferior wall MI, AV node damage, or toxic effects of drugs such as digoxin and propranolol.

Third-degree AV block occurring at the infranodal level is frequently associated with extensive anterior MI. It generally isn't the result of increases in parasympathetic tone or drug effect.

CLINICAL SIGNIFICANCE

Third-degree AV block occurring at the AV node, with a junctional escape rhythm, is usually transient and generally associated with a favorable prognosis. In third-degree AV block at the infranodal level, however, the pacemaker is unstable and episodes of ventricular asystole are common. The prognosis for third-degree AV block at this level is generally less favorable.

Because the ventricular rate in third-degree AV block can be slow and the decrease in cardiac output so significant, the arrhythmia usually results in a life-threatening situation. In addition, the loss of AV synchrony results in the loss of atrial kick, which further decreases cardiac output.

SIGNS AND SYMPTOMS

Most patients with third-degree AV block experience significant signs and symptoms, including severe fatigue, dyspnea, chest pain, light-headedness, changes in mental status, and changes in the level of consciousness. Hypotension, pallor, and diaphoresis may also occur. The peripheral pulse rate will be slow, but the rhythm will be regular.

A few patients will be relatively free of symptoms, complaining only that they can't tolerate exercise and that they're typically tired for no apparent reason. The severity of symptoms depends to a large extent on the resulting ventricular rate and the patient's ability to compensate for decreased cardiac output.

TREATMENT

If the patient is experiencing serious signs and symptoms related to the low heart rate, or if the patient's condition seems to be deteriorating, interventions may include transcu-

IDENTIFYING THIRD-DEGREE AV BLOCK

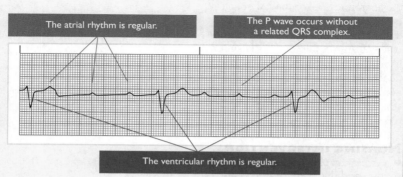

The atrial rhythm is regular.

The P wave occurs without a related QRS complex.

The ventricular rhythm is regular.

RHYTHM
◆ Atrial: Regular
◆ Ventricular: Regular

RATE
◆ Atrial: 60 to 100 beats/minute (atria act independently under control of sinoatrial node)
◆ Ventricular: Usually 40 to 60 beats/minute in an intranodal block (a junctional escape rhythm)
◆ Ventricular: Usually less than 40 beats/ minute in infranodal block (a ventricular escape rhythm)

P WAVE
◆ Normal size
◆ Normal configuration
◆ May be buried in QRS complex or T wave

PR INTERVAL
◆ Not measurable

QRS COMPLEX
◆ Configuration depends on location of escape mechanism and origin of ventricular depolarization
◆ Appears normal if the block is at the level of the atrioventricular (AV) node or bundle of His
◆ Widened if the block is at the level of the bundle branches

T WAVE
◆ Normal size
◆ Normal configuration
◆ May be abnormal if QRS complex originates in ventricle

QT INTERVAL
◆ Within normal limits

OTHER
◆ Atria and ventricles depolarized from different pacemaker sites and beat independently of each other
◆ P waves occur without QRS complexes

taneous pacing or I.V. dopamine or epinephrine.

Asymptomatic patients in third-degree AV block should be prepared for insertion of a transvenous temporary pacemaker until a decision is made about the need for a permanent pacemaker. If symptoms develop, a transcutaneous pacemaker should be used until the transvenous pacemaker is placed.

Because third-degree AV block occurring at the infranodal level is usually associated with extensive anterior MI, patients are more likely to have permanent third-degree AV block, which most likely requires insertion of a permanent pacemaker.

Third-degree AV block occurring at the anatomic level of the AV node can be caused by increased parasympathetic tone associated with an inferior wall MI. As a result, the block is more likely to be short-lived. In these patients, the decision to insert a permanent pacemaker is often delayed to assess how well the conduction system recovers.

NURSING INTERVENTIONS

- Assess the patient's tolerance of the rhythm and the need for interventions to improve cardiac output and relieve symptoms.
- Keep the patient on bed rest, if indicated, to reduce myocardial oxygen demand.
- Make sure that the patient has a patent I.V. line.
- Administer oxygen therapy, as ordered.
- Keep transcutaneous pacemaker at the bedside, as ordered.
- Teach the patient and family about the use of pacemakers if the patient requires one.

9

ELECTROLYTE DISTURBANCES

This chapter reviews electrocardiogram (ECG) characteristics associated with electrolyte disturbances.

Rhythm strips of patients with electrolyte disturbances such as hyperkalemia, hypokalemia, hypercalcemia, and hypocalcemia, commonly show distinctive patterns. By recognizing some of these variations early, you may be able to identify and treat potentially dangerous conditions before they become serious.

Remember though that the patient's ECG is only part of the clinical picture. Additional information such as the patient's medical history, findings on physical examination, and additional diagnostic studies are needed to confirm an initial diagnosis based on ECG analysis.

Potassium and calcium ions play a major role in the electrical activity of the heart. *Depolarization* results from the exchange of these ions across the cell membrane. Changes in ion concentration can affect the heart's electrical activity and, as a result, the patient's ECG. This section examines ECG effects from high and low potassium and calcium levels.

Hyperkalemia

Potassium, the most plentiful intracellular cation (positively charged electrolyte), contributes to many important cellular functions. Most of the body's potassium content is located in the cells. The intracellular fluid (ICF) concentration of potassium is 150 to 160 mEq/L; the extracellular fluid (ECF) concentration is 3.5 to 4.5 mEq/L. Many symptoms associated with potassium imbalance are caused by changes in this ratio of ICF to ECF potassium concentration. Hyperkalemia is generally defined as an elevation of potassium in the blood above 5 mEq/L.

CAUSES
Hyperkalemia can be caused by:
• an increased intake of potassium, including excessive dietary intake and I.V. administration of penicillin G, potassium supplements, or banked whole blood
• a shift of potassium from ICF to ECF occurring with changes in cell membrane permeability or damage,

ECG EFFECTS OF HYPERKALEMIA

The classic and most striking electrocardiogram (ECG) feature of hyperkalemia is tall, peaked T waves. This rhythm strip shows a typical peaked T wave (shaded area).

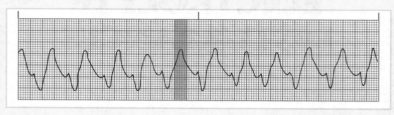

including extensive surgery, burns, massive crush injuries, cell hypoxia, acidosis, or insulin deficiency
● decreased renal excretion, including renal failure, decreased production and secretion of aldosterone, Addison's disease, and use of potassium-sparing diuretics.

CLINICAL SIGNIFICANCE

When extracellular potassium concentrations increase without a significant change in intracellular potassium concentrations, the cell becomes less negative, or partially depolarized, and the resting cell membrane potential decreases. Mild elevations in extracellular potassium result in cells that repolarize faster and are more irritable.

Alert More critical elevations in extracellular potassium result in an inability of cells to repolarize and respond to electrical stimuli. Cardiac standstill, or asystole, *is the most serious consequence of severe hyperkalemia.*

ECG CHARACTERISTICS

Rhythm: Atrial and ventricular rhythms are regular
Rate: Atrial and ventricular rates within normal limits

P wave: Low amplitude in mild hyperkalemia; wide and flattened P wave in moderate hyperkalemia; possible indiscernible P wave in severe hyperkalemia
PR interval: Normal or prolonged; not measurable if P wave can't be detected
QRS complex: Widened, because ventricular depolarization takes longer
ST segment: May be elevated in severe hyperkalemia
T wave: Tall, peaked; the classic and most striking feature of hyperkalemia
QT interval: Shortened
Other: Intraventricular conduction disturbances commonly occur (see *ECG effects of hyperkalemia*)

SIGNS AND SYMPTOMS

Mild hyperkalemia may cause neuromuscular irritability including restlessness, intestinal cramping, diarrhea, and tingling lips and fingers. Severe hyperkalemia may cause loss of muscle tone, muscle weakness, and paralysis.

INTERVENTIONS

Treatment depends on the severity of hyperkalemia and the patient's signs and symptoms. The underlying cause must be identified and the extracellular potassium concentration brought back to normal. Drug therapy to normalize potassium levels includes calcium gluconate to decrease neuromuscular irritability, insulin and glucose to facilitate the entry of potassium into the cell, and sodium bicarbonate to correct metabolic acidosis.

Oral or rectal administration of cation exchange resins, such as sodium polystyrene sulfonate, may be used to exchange sodium for potassium in the intestine. In the instance of renal failure or severe hyperkalemia, dialysis may be necessary to remove excess potassium. The patient's potassium blood levels should be monitored closely until they return to normal, and arrhythmias should be identified and managed appropriately.

Hypokalemia

Hypokalemia (potassium deficiency) occurs when the ECF concentration of potassium drops below 3.5 mEq/L, usually indicating a loss of total body potassium. The concentration of ECF potassium is so small that even minor changes in ECF potassium affect resting membrane potential.

CAUSES
Hypokalemia can be caused by:
- alcoholism, anorexia nervosa, and malnutrition
- an increased loss of body potassium, increased entry of potassium into cells, and reduced potassium intake. (Shifts in potassium from the extracellular space to the intracellular space may be caused by alkalosis, especially respiratory alkalosis. Intracellular uptake of potassium is also increased by catecholamines.)

- dietary deficiencies in elderly patients (rarely occurs).
- GI and renal disorders — most commonly cause potassium loss from body stores. (GI losses of potassium are associated with laxative abuse, intestinal fistulae or drainage tubes, diarrhea, vomiting, and continuous nasogastric drainage. Renal loss of potassium is related to increased secretion of potassium by the distal tubule. Diuretics, a low magnesium concentration in the blood, and excessive aldosterone secretion may cause urinary loss of potassium.)
- several antibiotics, including gentamicin and amphotericin B.

CLINICAL SIGNIFICANCE
When extracellular potassium levels decrease rapidly and intracellular potassium concentration doesn't change, the resting membrane potential becomes more negative and the cell membrane becomes hyperpolarized. The cardiac effects of hypokalemia are related to these changes in membrane excitability. Ventricular repolarization is delayed because potassium contributes to the repolarization phase of the action potential.

Alert *Hypokalemia can cause dangerous ventricular arrhythmias and increase the risk of digoxin toxicity.*

ECG CHARACTERISTICS
Rhythm: Atrial and ventricular rhythms regular
Rate: Atrial and ventricular rates within normal limits
P wave: Usually normal size and configuration, but may become peaked in severe hypokalemia
PR interval: May be prolonged
QRS complex: Within normal limits or possibly widened; prolonged in severe hypokalemia

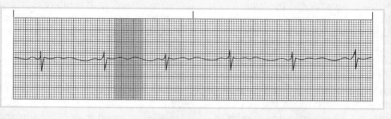

ECG EFFECTS OF HYPOKALEMIA

As the potassium concentration in the blood drops, the T wave becomes flat and a U wave appears (shaded area). This rhythm strip shows typical electrocardiogram (ECG) effects of hypokalemia.

QT interval: Usually indiscernible as the T wave flattens

ST segment: Depressed

T wave: Decreased amplitude (The T wave becomes flat as the potassium level drops. In severe hypokalemia, it flattens completely and may become inverted. The T wave also may fuse with an increasingly prominent U wave.)

Other: Increased amplitude of U wave, becomes more prominent as hypokalemia worsens and fuses with T wave (see *ECG effects of hypokalemia*)

SIGNS AND SYMPTOMS

The most common symptoms of hypokalemia are caused by neuromuscular and cardiac effects, including smooth muscle atony, skeletal muscle weakness, and cardiac arrhythmias. Loss of smooth muscle tone results in constipation, intestinal distention, nausea, vomiting, anorexia, and paralytic ileus.

Alert In hypokalemia, skeletal muscle weakness occurs first in the larger muscles of the arms and legs and eventually affects the diaphragm, causing respiratory arrest.

Cardiac effects of hypokalemia include arrhythmias, such as bradycardia, atrioventricular (AV) block, and ventricular arrhythmias. Delayed depolarization leads to characteristic changes on the ECG.

INTERVENTIONS

The underlying causes of hypokalemia should be identified and corrected. Correct acid-base imbalances, replace potassium losses, and prevent further losses. Encourage intake of foods and fluids rich in potassium. Oral or I.V. potassium supplements may be administered. Monitor the patient's potassium blood levels until they return to normal, and identify cardiac arrhythmias and manage them appropriately.

Hypercalcemia

Most of the body's calcium stores (99%) are located in bone. The remainder is found in the plasma and body cells. About 50% of plasma calcium is bound to plasma proteins. About 40% is found in the ionized or free form.

Calcium plays an important role in myocardial contractility. Ionized calcium is more important than plasma-

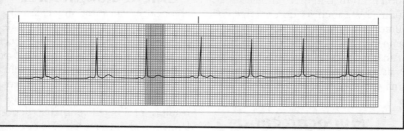

ECG EFFECTS OF HYPERCALCEMIA

Increased concentrations of calcium in the blood cause shortening of the QT interval as shown (shaded area) in this electrocardiogram (ECG) rhythm strip.

bound calcium in physiologic functions. Hypercalcemia is usually defined as a serum calcium concentration greater than 10.5 mg/dl.

CAUSES

The causes of hypercalcemia include:
- bone metastasis and calcium resorption associated with cancers of the breast, prostate, and cervix
- excess vitamin D intake
- hyperparathyroidism
- parathyroid hormone–producing tumors
- sarcoidosis
- certain drugs such as lithium.

CLINICAL SIGNIFICANCE

In hypercalcemia, calcium is found inside cells in excess amounts. The cell membrane becomes refractory to depolarization as a result of a more positive action potential. This loss of cell membrane excitability causes many of the cardiac symptoms in patients with hypercalcemia.

Both ventricular depolarization and repolarization are accelerated. The patient may experience bradyarrhythmias and varying degrees of AV block.

ECG CHARACTERISTICS

Rhythm: Atrial and ventricular rhythms regular

Rate: Atrial and ventricular rates within normal limits, but bradycardia can occur

P wave: Normal size and configuration

PR interval: May be prolonged

QRS complex: Within normal limits, but may be prolonged

QT interval: Shortened

ST segment: Shortened

T wave: Normal size and configuration; may be depressed

Other: None (see *ECG effects of hypercalcemia*)

SIGNS AND SYMPTOMS

Common signs and symptoms of hypercalcemia include anorexia, nausea, constipation, lethargy, fatigue, and weakness. Behavioral changes also may occur. Renal calculi may form as precipitates of calcium salts, and impaired renal function is common. A reciprocal decrease in phosphate levels in the blood often accompanies elevated levels of calcium in the blood.

INTERVENTIONS

Treatment of hypercalcemia focuses on identifying and managing the underlying cause and is guided by the severity of the patient's symptoms. Administration of oral phosphate is usually effective as long as renal function is normal. In more critical situations, I.V. administration of large volumes of normal saline solution may enhance renal excretion of calcium. Patients in renal failure may need dialysis. Corticosteroids and calcitonin may be used to treat hypercalcemia.

Hypocalcemia

Hypocalcemia occurs when the calcium level in the blood falls below 8.5 mg/dl.

CAUSES

The causes of hypocalcemia include:
- citrate solution — used in storing whole blood, binding with calcium
- decreased intestinal absorption of calcium caused by vitamin D deficiency, either from inadequate vitamin D intake or insufficient exposure to sunlight
- decreases in parathyroid hormone and vitamin D, inadequate intestinal absorption, blood administration, or deposition of ionized calcium into soft tissue or bone
- excessive dietary intake of phosphorus that binds with calcium and prevents calcium absorption
- inadequate dietary intake of green, leafy vegetables or dairy products — causing a nutritional deficiency of calcium
- malabsorption of fats, removal of the parathyroid glands, metabolic or respiratory alkalosis, and hypo-albuminemia

- pancreatitis (decreases ionized calcium) or neoplastic bone metastases (decreases serum calcium levels).

CLINICAL SIGNIFICANCE

Hypocalcemia causes an increase in neuromuscular excitability. Partial depolarization of nerves and muscle cells result from a decrease in threshold potential. As a result, a smaller stimulus is needed to initiate an action potential. Characteristic ECG changes are a result of prolonged ventricular depolarization and decreased cardiac contractility.

ECG CHARACTERISTICS

Rhythm: Atrial and ventricular rhythms regular
Rate: Atrial and ventricular rates within normal limits
P wave: Normal size and configuration
PR interval: Within normal limits
QRS complex: Within normal limits
QT interval: Prolonged
ST segment: Prolonged
T wave: Normal size and configuration, but may become flat or inverted
Other: None (see *ECG effects of hypocalcemia*)

SIGNS AND SYMPTOMS

Signs and symptoms of hypocalcemia include hyperreflexia, carpopedal spasm, confusion, and circumoral and digital paresthesia. Hyperactive bowel sounds and intestinal cramping may also occur.

Alert *In hypocalcemia, severe symptoms include tetany, seizures, and respiratory arrest, which may lead to death. Clinical signs that indicate hypocalcemia include Trousseau's sign and Chvostek's sign.*

ECG EFFECTS OF HYPOCALCEMIA

Decreased concentrations of calcium in the blood prolong the QT interval, as shown (shaded area) in this electrocardiogram (ECG) rhythm strip.

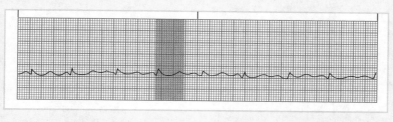

INTERVENTIONS

Treatment should focus on identifying and managing the underlying causes of hypocalcemia. Severe signs and symptoms require emergency treatment with I.V. calcium gluconate. Monitor serum calcium levels and replace oral calcium when possible. Cardiac arrhythmias need to be identified and managed appropriately. Long-term management of hypocalcemia includes decreasing phosphate intake.

PART 3

◆

Interpreting 12-lead ECGs

NORMAL 12-LEAD ECG

The 12-lead electrocardiogram (ECG) is a diagnostic test that helps identify pathologic conditions, especially ischemia and acute myocardial infarction (MI). It provides a more complete view of the heart's electrical activity than does a rhythm strip, and can be used to assess left ventricular function more effectively. Patients with conditions that affect the heart's electrical system may also benefit from a 12-lead ECG, including those with:

- cardiac arrhythmias
- digoxin or other drug toxicity
- electrolyte imbalances
- heart chamber enlargement or hypertrophy
- hypothermia
- pacemakers
- pericarditis
- pulmonary embolism.

Like other diagnostic tests, a 12-lead ECG must be viewed in conjunction with other clinical data. Always correlate the patient's ECG results with the history, physical assessment findings, and results of laboratory and other diagnostic studies as well as the drug regimen.

The 12-lead ECG records the heart's electrical activity using a series of electrodes placed on the patient's extremities and chest wall. The 12 leads include three bipolar limb leads (I, II, and III), three unipolar augmented limb leads (aV_R, aV_L, and aV_F), and six unipolar precordial, or chest, leads (V_1, V_2, V_3, V_4, V_5, and V_6). These leads provide 12 different views of the heart's electrical activity. (See *Viewing ECG leads,* page 136.)

Scanning up, down, and across, each lead transmits information about a different area of the heart. The waveforms obtained from each lead vary depending on the lead's location in relation to the wave of depolarization passing through the myocardium.

LIMB LEADS

The six limb leads record electrical activity in the heart's frontal plane, a view through the middle of the heart from top to bottom and right to left.

PRECORDIAL LEADS

The six precordial leads provide information on electrical activity in the heart's horizontal plane, a transverse view through the middle of the heart, dividing it into upper and lower portions.

ELECTRICAL AXES

As well as assessing 12 different leads, a 12-lead ECG records the heart's

VIEWING ECG LEADS

Each of the leads on a 12-lead electrocardiogram (ECG) views the heart from a different angle. These illustrations show the direction of electrical activity (depolarization) monitored by each lead and the corresponding 12 views of the heart.

VIEWS REFLECTED ON A 12-LEAD ECG	LEAD	VIEW OF THE HEART
	Standard limb leads (bipolar)	
	I	Lateral wall
	II	Inferior wall
	III	Inferior wall
	Augmented limb leads (unipolar)	
	aV$_R$	No specific view
	aV$_L$	Lateral wall
	aV$_F$	Inferior wall
	Precordial, or chest, leads (unipolar)	
	V$_1$	Septal wall
	V$_2$	Septal wall
	V$_3$	Anterior wall
	V$_4$	Anterior wall
	V$_5$	Lateral wall
	V$_6$	Lateral wall

electrical axis. The term *axis* refers to the direction of depolarization as it spreads through the heart. As impulses travel through the heart, they generate small electrical forces called *instantaneous vectors*. The mean of these vectors represents the force and direc-

tion of the wave of depolarization through the heart—the electrical axis. The electrical axis is also called the *mean instantaneous vector* or the *mean QRS vector*.

In a healthy heart, impulses originate in the sinoatrial node, travel through the atria to the atrioventricular node, and then travel to the ventricles. Most of the movement of the impulses is downward and to the left, the direction of a normal axis.

In an unhealthy heart, axis direction varies. That's because the direction of electrical activity travels away from areas of damage or necrosis, and toward areas of hypertrophy. Knowing the normal deflection of each lead will help you evaluate whether the electrical axis is normal or abnormal.

Obtaining a 12-lead ECG

To conduct a 12-lead ECG, you'll need to prepare properly, select the appropriate electrode sites, understand how to perform variations on a standard 12-lead ECG, and make an accurate recording.

PREPARATION

Gather all necessary supplies, including the ECG machine, recording paper, electrodes, and gauze pads. Tell the patient that the practitioner has ordered an ECG, and explain the procedure. Emphasize that the test takes about 10 minutes and that it's a safe and painless way to evaluate the heart's electrical activity. Answer the patient's questions, and offer reassurance. Preparing the patient properly will help alleviate anxiety and promote cooperation.

Ask the patient to lie flat in the center of the bed with his arms at his sides. If he can't tolerate lying flat, raise the head of the bed to the semi-Fowler's position. Document the patient's position during the procedure. Ensure privacy, and expose the patient's arms, legs, and chest, draping for comfort.

SITE SELECTION

Select the areas where you'll apply the electrodes. Choose areas that are flat and fleshy, not muscular or bony. Clip excessive hair from the area. Remove excess oil and other substances (such as body lotion) from the skin to improve electrode contact. Remember, better electrode contact results in better recording.

The 12-lead ECG provides 12 different views of the heart, just as 12 photographers snapping the same picture from different angles would produce 12 different photographs. Taking all of those snapshots requires placing four electrodes on the limbs and six across the front of the chest wall.

To help ensure an accurate recording, the electrodes must be applied correctly. Inaccurate placement of an electrode by more than $3/5''$ (1.5 cm) from its standard position may lead to inaccurate waveforms and an incorrect ECG interpretation.

You'll need patience when obtaining a pediatric ECG. With parental help, if possible, try distracting the child 's attention. If artifact from arm and leg movement is a problem, try placing the electrodes in a more proximal position on the extremity.

Limb lead placement

To record the bipolar limb leads I, II, and III and the unipolar limb leads aV_R, aV_L, and aV_F, place electrodes on both of the patient's arms and on his left leg. The right leg also receives an electrode, but that electrode acts as a ground and doesn't contribute to the waveform. (See *Limb lead placement*, pages 138 and 139.)

(Text continues on page 140.)

LIMB LEAD PLACEMENT

Proper lead placement is critical for accurate recording of cardiac rhythms. These diagrams show electrode placement for the six limb leads. RA indicates right arm; LA, left arm; RL, right leg; and LL, left leg. The plus sign (+) indicates the positive pole, the minus sign (−) indicates the negative pole, and G indicates the ground. To the left of each diagram is a sample electrocardiogram recording for that lead.

LEAD I
Connects the right arm (negative pole) with the left arm (positive pole)

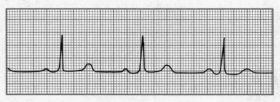
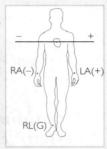

LEAD II
Connects the right arm (negative pole) with the left leg (positive pole)

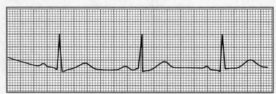
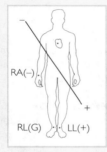

LEAD III
Connects the left arm (negative pole) with the left leg (positive pole)

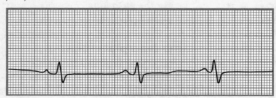
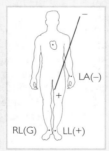

LEAD aV$_R$
Connects the right arm (positive pole) with the heart (negative pole)

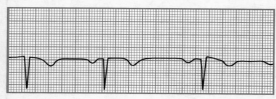
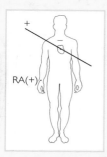

LEAD aV$_L$
Connects the left arm (positive pole) with the heart (negative pole)

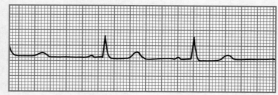
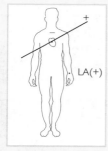

LEAD aV$_F$
Connects the left leg (positive pole) with the heart (negative pole)

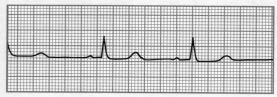
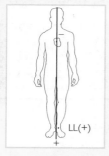

PRECORDIAL LEAD PLACEMENT

The precordial leads complement the limb leads to provide a complete view of the heart. To record the precordial leads, place the electrodes as shown.

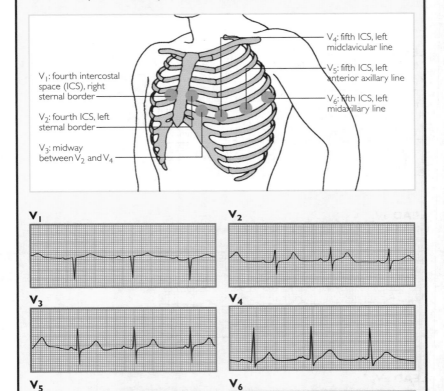

V_1: fourth intercostal space (ICS), right sternal border

V_2: fourth ICS, left sternal border

V_3: midway between V_2 and V_4

V_4: fifth ICS, left midclavicular line

V_5: fifth ICS, left anterior axillary line

V_6: fifth ICS, left midaxillary line

V_1

V_2

V_3

V_4

V_5

V_6

Placing the electrodes on the patient is typically easy because each leadwire is labeled or color-coded. For example, a wire (usually white) might be labeled "RA" for right arm. Another (usually red) might be labeled "LL" for left leg.

Precordial lead placement

Precordial leads are also labeled or color-coded according to which wire corresponds to which lead. To record the six precordial leads (V_1 through V_6), position the electrodes on specific areas of the anterior chest wall. (See *Precordial lead placement*.) If they're placed too low or too high, the ECG tracing will be inaccurate.

- Place lead V_1 over the fourth intercostal space (ICS) at the right sternal border. To find the space, locate the sternal notch at the second rib and feel your way down the sternal border until you reach the fourth ICS.
- Place lead V_2 just opposite V_1, over the fourth ICS at the left sternal border.
- Place lead V_4 over the fifth ICS at the left midclavicular line. Placing lead V_4 before V_3 makes it easier to see where to place lead V_3.
- Place lead V_3 midway between V_2 and V_4.
- Place lead V_5 over the fifth ICS at the left anterior axillary line.
- Place lead V_6 over the fifth ICS at the left midaxillary line. If you've placed leads V_4 through V_6 correctly, they should line up horizontally.

ADDITIONAL TYPES OF ECG LEADS

In addition to the standard 12-lead ECG, two other types of ECG leads may be used for diagnostic purposes: the posterior-lead ECG and the right chest–lead ECG. These ECG leads use chest and posterior leads to assess areas that standard 12-lead ECGs can't.

Posterior-lead ECG

Because of lung and muscle barriers, the usual chest leads can't "see" the heart's posterior surface to record myocardial damage there. To compensate for this, some practitioners add three posterior leads to the 12-lead ECG: leads V_7, V_8, and V_9. These leads are placed opposite anterior leads V_4, V_5, and V_6, on the left side of the patient's back, following the same horizontal line. (See *Posterior lead placement,* page 142.)

Occasionally, a physician may request right-sided posterior leads. These leads are labeled V_{7R}, V_{8R}, and V_{9R} and are placed on the right side of the patient's back. Their placement is a mirror image of the electrodes on the left side of the back. This type of ECG provides information on the right posterior area of the heart.

Right chest–lead ECG

The standard 12-lead ECG evaluates only the left ventricle. If the right ventricle needs to be assessed for damage or dysfunction, the physician may order a right chest–lead ECG. For example, a patient with an inferior wall MI might have a right chest–lead ECG to rule out right ventricular involvement.

With this type of ECG, the six leads are placed on the right side of the chest in a mirror image of the standard precordial lead placement. Electrodes start at the left sternal border and swing down under the right breast area. (See *Right precordial lead placement,* page 143.)

RECORDING THE ECG

After properly placing the electrodes, record the ECG. ECG machines come in two types: multichannel recorders (most common) and single-channel recorders. With a multichannel recorder, all electrodes are attached to the patient at once and the machine prints a simultaneous view of all leads. With a single-channel recorder, one lead at a time is recorded in a short strip by attaching and removing electrodes and stopping and starting the tracing each time. (See *Normal findings in a 12-lead ECG,* pages 144 to 146.)

To record a multichannel ECG, follow these steps:

POSTERIOR LEAD PLACEMENT

Posterior leads can be used to assess the heart's posterior surface. To ensure an accurate reading, make sure the posterior electrodes V_7, V_8, and V_9 are placed at the same horizontal level as the V_6 lead at the fifth intercostal space. Place lead V_7 at the posterior axillary line, lead V_9 at the paraspinal line, and lead V_8 halfway between leads V_7 and V_9.

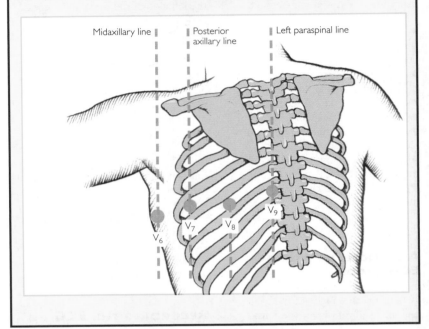

- Plug the cord of the ECG machine into a grounded outlet. If the machine operates on a charged battery, it may not need to be plugged in.
- Place all of the electrodes on the patient.
- Make sure all leads are securely attached, and then turn on the machine.
- To prevent distortion of the ECG tracing, instruct the patient to relax, lie still, breathe normally, and avoid talking during the recording.
- Set the ECG paper speed selector to 25 mm/second. If necessary, enter the patient's identification data.

- Press the appropriate button on the ECG machine and record the ECG.
- Observe the quality of the tracing. When the machine finishes the recording, turn it off.
- Remove the electrodes and clean the patient's skin.

ECG PRINTOUT

Depending on the information entered, ECG printouts from a multichannel ECG machine will show the patient's name, birth date, and medical record number. At the top of the printout, you'll see the patient's heart rate and wave durations, measured in

RIGHT PRECORDIAL LEAD PLACEMENT

Right precordial leads can provide specific information about the function of the right ventricle. Place the six leads on the right side of the chest in a mirror image of the standard precordial lead placement, as shown here.

V_{1R}: fourth intercostal space (ICS), left sternal border
V_{2R}: fourth ICS, right sternal border
V_{3R}: halfway between V_{2R} and V_{4R}
V_{4R}: fifth ICS, right midclavicular line
V_{5R}: fifth ICS, right anterior axillary line
V_{6R}: fifth ICS, right midaxillary line

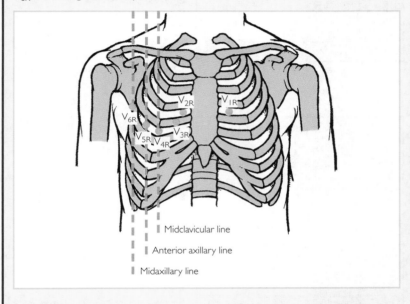

Midclavicular line

Anterior axillary line

Midaxillary line

seconds. (See *Reading the multichannel ECG recording,* page 147.)

Some machines can record ST-segment elevation and depression. The name of the lead will appear next to each 6-second strip.

If it isn't already included on the printout, be sure to write the following information: date, time, physician's name, and special circumstances. For example, you might record an episode of chest pain, ab-

normal electrolyte levels, related drug treatment, abnormal placement of the electrodes, presence of an artificial pacemaker, and whether a magnet was used (to disable a pacemaker) while the ECG was obtained.

Remember, ECGs are legal documents. They belong in the patient's medical record and must be saved for future reference and comparison with baseline strips.

Normal findings in a 12-lead ECG

Each electrocardiogram (ECG) waveform (P wave, QRS complex, T wave) represents the electrical events that occur during one cardiac cycle. The 12-lead ECG provides 12 views of the electrical activity of the heart, which includes three bipolar leads (I, II, and III), three unipolar augmented leads (aV$_R$, aV$_L$, and aV$_F$), and six precordial, or chest leads (V$_1$, V$_2$, V$_3$, V$_4$, V$_5$, and V$_6$). Each lead on a 12-lead ECG views the heart from a different angle. The tracings shown here represent normal findings of the heart's electrical activity in each of the 12 leads.

LEAD I

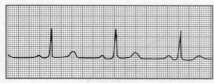

P wave: Upright
Q wave: Small or none
R wave: Largest wave
S wave: None present, or smaller than R wave
T wave: Upright
U wave: None present
ST segment: Usually isoelectric, but may vary from +1 to –0.5 mm

LEAD II

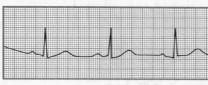

P wave: Upright
Q wave: Small or none
R wave: Large (vertical heart)
S wave: None present, or smaller than R wave
T wave: Upright
U wave: None present
ST segment: Usually isoelectric, but may vary from +1 to –0.5 mm

LEAD III

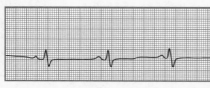

P wave: Upright, diphasic, or inverted
Q wave: Usually small or none (a Q wave must also be present in lead aV$_F$ to be considered diagnostic)
R wave: None present to large wave
S wave: None present to large wave, indicating horizontal heart
T wave: Upright, diphasic, or inverted
U wave: None present
ST segment: Usually isoelectric, but may vary from +1 to –0.5 mm

LEAD aV$_R$

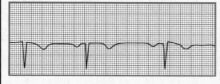

P wave: Inverted
Q wave: None, small wave, or large wave present
R wave: None, or small wave present
S wave: Large wave (may be QS)
T wave: Inverted
U wave: None present
ST segment: Usually isoelectric, but may vary from +1 to –0.5 mm

LEAD aV_L

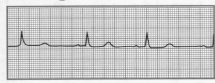

P wave: Upright, diphasic, or inverted
Q wave: None, small wave, or large wave present (a Q wave must also be present in lead I or precordial leads to be considered diagnostic)
R wave: None, small wave, or large wave present (large wave indicates horizontal heart)
S wave: None present to large wave (large wave indicates vertical heart)
T wave: Upright, diphasic, or inverted
U wave: None present
ST segment: Usually isoelectric, but may vary from +1 to –0.5 mm

LEAD aV_F

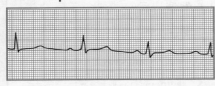

P wave: Upright
Q wave: None, or small wave present
R wave: None, small wave, or large wave present (large wave suggests vertical heart)
S wave: None present to large wave (large wave suggests horizontal heart)
T wave: Upright, diphasic, or inverted
U wave: None present
ST segment: Usually isoelectric, but may vary from +1 to –0.5 mm

LEAD V_1

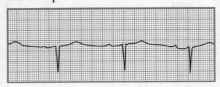

P wave: Upright, diphasic, or inverted
Q wave: Deep QS pattern possibly present
R wave: None present, or less than S wave
S wave: Large (part of QS pattern)
T wave: Usually inverted, but may be upright and diphasic
U wave: None present
ST segment: May vary from 0 to +1 mm

LEAD V_2

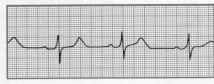

P wave: Upright
Q wave: Deep QS pattern possibly present
R wave: None present, or less than S wave (wave may become progressively larger)
S wave: Large (part of QS pattern)
T wave: Upright
U wave: Upright; lower amplitude than T wave
ST segment: May vary from 0 to +1mm

(continued)

LEAD V₃

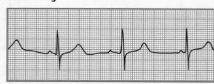

P wave: Upright
Q wave: None, or small wave present
R wave: Less than, greater than, or equal to S wave (wave may become progressively larger)
S wave: Large (greater than R wave, less than R wave, or equal to R wave)
T wave: Upright
U wave: Upright; lower amplitude than T wave
ST segment: May vary from 0 to +1 mm

LEAD V₄

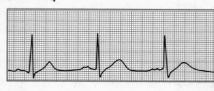

P wave: Upright
Q wave: None, or small wave present
R wave: Progressively larger wave; R wave greater than S wave
S wave: Progressively smaller (less than R wave)
T wave: Upright
U wave: Upright; lower amplitude than T wave
ST segment: Usually isoelectric, but may vary from +1 to −0.5 mm

LEAD V₅

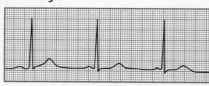

P wave: Upright
Q wave: Small
R wave: Progressively larger, but less than 26 mm
S wave: Progressively smaller; less than the S wave in V₄
T wave: Upright
U wave: None present
ST segment: Usually isoelectric, but may vary from +1 to −0.5 mm

LEAD V₆

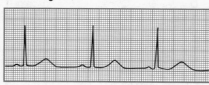

P wave: Upright
Q wave: Small
R wave: Largest wave, but less than 26 mm
S wave: Smallest wave; less than the S wave in V₅
T wave: Upright
U wave: None present
ST segment: Usually isoelectric, but may vary from +1 to −0.5 mm

READING THE MULTICHANNEL ECG RECORDING

The top of a 12-lead electrocardiogram (ECG) recording usually shows patient identification information along with an interpretation by the machine. A rhythm strip is commonly included at the bottom of the recording.

STANDARDIZATION

Look for standardization marks on the recording, normally 10 small squares high. If the patient has high voltage complexes, the marks will be half as high. You'll also notice that lead markers separate the lead recordings on the paper and that each lead is labeled.

Familiarize yourself with the order in which the leads are arranged on an ECG tracing. Getting accustomed to the layout of the tracing will help you interpret the ECG more quickly and accurately.

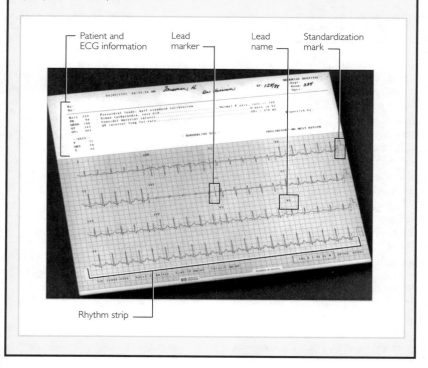

Patient and ECG information   Lead marker   Lead name   Standardization mark

Rhythm strip

ELECTRICAL AXIS DETERMINATION

Electrical axis

The *electrical axis* is the average direction of the heart's electrical activity during ventricular depolarization. Leads placed on the body sense the sum of the heart's electrical activity and record it as waveforms.

You can determine your patient's electrical axis by examining the waveforms recorded from the six frontal plane leads: I, II, III, aV_R, aV_L, and aV_F. Imaginary lines drawn from each of the leads intersect at the center of the heart and form a diagram known as the hexaxial reference system. (See *Understanding the hexaxial reference system.*)

An axis that falls between 0 and 90 degrees is considered normal (some sources consider –30 to 90-degrees to be normal). An axis between 90 and 180 degrees indicates right axis deviation, and one between 0 and –90 degrees indicates left axis deviation (some sources consider –30 to –90 degrees to be left axis deviation). An axis between –180 and –90 degrees indicates extreme right axis deviation and is called an indeterminate axis.

In the neonate, right axis deviation, between +60 and +160 degrees, is normal because of the dominance of the right ventricle. By age 1, the axis shifts to fall between +10 and +100 degrees as the left ventricle becomes dominant.

In elderly patients, left axis deviation commonly occurs. This axis shift may be caused by fibrosis of the anterior fascicle of the left bundle branch, and because the thickness of the left ventricular wall increases by 25% between ages 30 and 80.

ELECTRICAL AXIS DETERMINATION

To determine your patient's electrical axis, use the *quadrant method* or the *degree method.*

Quadrant method

The quadrant method—a fast, easy way to plot the heart's axis—involves observing the main deflection of the QRS complex in leads I and aV_F. (See *Using the quadrant method,* page 150.) Lead I indicates whether impulses are moving to the right or left, and lead aV_F indicates whether they're moving up or down.

If the QRS-complex deflection is positive or upright in both leads, the

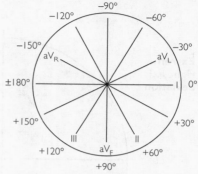
electrical axis is normal. If lead I is upright and lead aV$_F$ points down, left axis deviation exists.

When lead I points down and lead aV$_F$ is upright, right axis deviation exists. Both waves pointing down indicates extreme right axis deviation.

Degree method

The degree method is a more precise axis calculation that provides an exact measurement of the electrical axis. (See *Using the degree method,* page 151.) It also allows you to determine the axis even if the QRS complex isn't clearly positive or negative in leads I and aV$_F$. To use this method, follow these four steps:

● Review all six limb leads, and identify the one that contains either the smallest QRS complex or the complex with an equal deflection above and below the baseline.

● Use the hexaxial diagram to identify the lead perpendicular to this lead. For example, if lead I has the smallest QRS complex, then the lead perpendicular to the line representing lead I would be lead aV$_F$.

● After you've identified the perpendicular lead, examine its QRS complex. If the electrical activity is moving toward the positive pole of a lead, the QRS complex deflects upward. If it's moving away from the positive pole of a lead, the QRS complex deflects downward.

● Plot this information on the hexaxial diagram to determine the direction of the electrical axis.

AXIS DEVIATION

Finding a patient's electrical axis can help confirm a diagnosis or narrow the range of possible diagnoses. Factors that influence the location of the axis include the heart's position in the chest, the heart's size, the patient's body size or type, the conduction pathways, and the force of the electrical impulses that is generated.

USING THE QUADRANT METHOD

This chart will help you quickly determine the direction of a patient's electrical axis. Observe the deflections of the QRS complexes in leads I and aV_F. Then check the chart to determine whether the patient's axis is normal or has a left, right, or extreme right axis deviation.

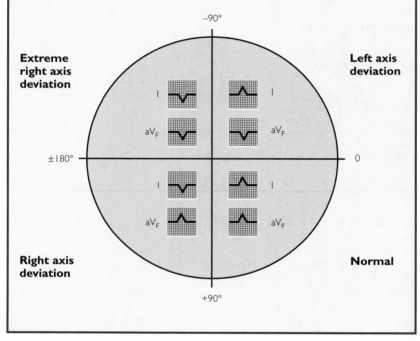

Causes of *left axis deviation* include:
- aging
- aortic stenosis
- inferior wall myocardial infarction (MI)
- left anterior hemiblock
- left bundle-branch block
- left ventricular hypertrophy
- mechanical shifts (ascites, pregnancy, tumors)
- normal variation
- Wolff-Parkinson-White syndrome.

Causes of *right axis deviation* include:
- emphysema
- lateral wall MI
- left posterior hemiblock
- normal variation
- pulmonary hypertension
- pulmonic stenosis
- right bundle-branch block (RBBB)
- right ventricular hypertrophy.

Remember that electrical activity in the heart swings away from areas of damage or necrosis, so the damaged part of the heart will be the last area depolarized. For example, in RBBB, the impulse travels quickly down the normal left side and then moves slowly down the right side. This shifts the electrical forces to the right, causing right axis deviation.

USING THE DEGREE METHOD

The degree method of determining axis deviation allows you to identify a patient's electrical axis by degrees on the hexaxial system, not just by quadrant. To use this method, take the following steps.

STEP 1

Identify the limb lead with the smallest QRS complex or the equiphasic QRS complex. In this example, it's lead III.

LEAD I

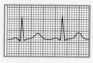

LEAD II

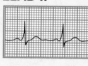

LEAD III

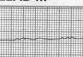

LEAD aV$_R$

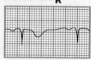

LEAD aV$_L$

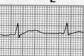

LEAD aV$_F$

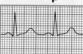

STEP 2

Locate the axis for lead III on the hexaxial diagram. Then find the axis perpendicular to it, which is the axis for lead aV$_R$.

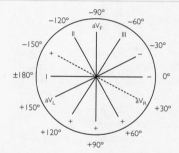

STEP 3

Now, examine the QRS complex in lead aV$_R$, noting whether the deflection is positive or negative. As you can see, the QRS complex for this lead is negative, indicating that the current is moving toward the negative pole of aV$_R$, which is in the right lower quadrant at +30 degrees on the hexaxial diagram. So the electrical axis here is normal at +30 degrees.

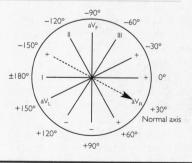

Axis deviation isn't always clinically significant, and it isn't always cardiac in origin. For example, infants and children typically have right axis deviation. Pregnant women typically have left axis deviation.

12

ACUTE CORONARY SYNDROMES

A 12-lead electrocardiogram (ECG) is used to assist in the diagnosis of certain conditions such as unstable angina, myocardial infarction (MI), and pericarditis. By reviewing sample ECGs, you'll know the classic signs to look for. This chapter examines ECG characteristics of each of these cardiac conditions.

Acute MI (ST-segment elevation MI [STEMI] and non–ST-segment elevation MI [NSTEMI]) and unstable angina are now recognized as part of a group of clinical diseases called *acute coronary syndromes* (ACSs).

Rupture or erosion of plaque—an unstable and lipid-rich substance—starts all coronary syndromes. The rupture causes platelet adhesions, fibrin clot formation, and activation of thrombin. (See *Understanding thrombus formation.*)

Early thrombus doesn't necessarily block coronary blood flow. When the thrombus does progress and occludes blood flow, an ACS results.

The degree of blockage and the time that the affected vessel remains occluded are major factors in the type of infarct that occurs.

For patients with unstable angina, a thrombus partially occludes a coronary vessel. This thrombus is full of platelets. The partially occluded vessel may have distal microthrombi that cause necrosis in some myocytes. These patients may progress to a non–ST-segment elevation MI.

A thrombus that fully occludes the vessel for a prolonged time is known as an *ST-segment elevation MI*. In this type of MI, there's a greater concentration of thrombin and fibrin.

CAUSES OF ACS

Causes of ACS include atherosclerosis and embolus. In atherosclerosis, plaque forms and subsequently ruptures or erodes, resulting in platelet adhesions, fibrin clot formation, and activation of thrombin.

Risk factors for ACS include:
- diabetes
- dyslipidemia
- family history of heart disease
- high-fat, high-carbohydrate diet
- hypertension
- inflammation
- menopause
- obesity
- sedentary lifestyle
- smoking
- stress.

UNDERSTANDING THROMBUS FORMATION

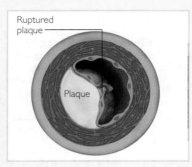

1. Plaque in coronary artery ruptures or erodes.

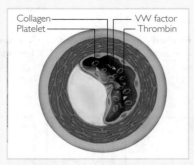

2. Platelets adhere to damaged area and become exposed to activating factors (collagen, thrombin, von Willebrand [VW] factor).

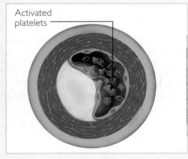

3. Platelet activation produces glycoprotein IIb and IIIa receptors that bind fibrinogen.

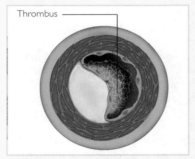

4. Platelet aggregation and adhesion continue, enlarging thrombus.

SIGNS AND SYMPTOMS
Angina

A patient with *angina* typically experiences burning, squeezing, or crushing tightness in the substernal or precordial chest that may radiate to the left arm, neck, jaw, or shoulder blade.

Angina usually follows physical exertion, but also may occur after emotional excitement, exposure to temperature extremes, or a large meal. Angina has four major forms, although only unstable angina is classified as an ACS.

- *Stable angina*—pain is predictable in frequency and duration, and it can be relieved with nitroglycerin and rest.
- *Unstable angina*—pain increases in frequency and duration and is more easily induced, which indicates a worsening of coronary artery disease. This may progress to MI.
- *Prinzmetal* (or *variant*) *angina*—pain is caused by unpredictable spasm of the coronary arteries that may occur

ECG CHANGES ASSOCIATED WITH ANGINA

Illustrated below are some classic electrocardiogram (ECG) changes involving the T wave and ST segment that you may see when monitoring a patient with angina.

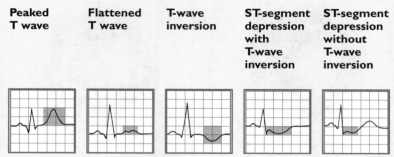

| Peaked T wave | Flattened T wave | T-wave inversion | ST-segment depression with T-wave inversion | ST-segment depression without T-wave inversion |

spontaneously; it may not be related to physical exercise or emotional stress.

● *Microvascular angina*—angina-like pain caused by impairment of vaso-dilator reserve in a patient with normal coronary arteries.

MI

Although other diagnoses may have chest pain as a symptom, retrosternal chest discomfort, pain, or pressure is a prime symptom of an infarction.

Patients typically describe these symptoms of acute ischemia and MI:
● uncomfortable pressure, squeezing, burning, severe persistent pain, or fullness in the center of the chest lasting several minutes (usually longer than 15 minutes)
● pain radiating to the shoulders, neck, arms, or jaws, or pain in the back between the shoulder blades
● accompanying symptoms of lightheadedness, fainting, sweating, nausea, shortness of breath, anxiety, or a feeling of impending doom.

Most patients experience typical chest pain with acute ischemia and

MI; but women, and occasionally men, elderly patients, and patients with diabetes, may experience atypical chest pain. Atypical symptoms include upper back discomfort between the shoulder blades, palpitations, a feeling of fullness in the neck, nausea, abdominal discomfort, dizziness, unexplained fatigue, and exhaustion or shortness of breath.

ECG CHARACTERISTICS
Angina

● Most patients with angina show ischemic changes on an ECG only during the attack. (See *ECG changes associated with angina*.) Because these changes may be fleeting, always obtain an order to perform a 12-lead ECG as soon as the patient reports chest pain. When necessary, perform additional posterior and right precordial ECG leads.
● The ECG may help you determine which area of the heart and which coronary arteries are involved. By recognizing danger early, you may be able to prevent MI or even death. (See *Identifying Wellens syndrome*.)

IDENTIFYING WELLENS SYNDROME

Wellens syndrome occurs in about 14% to 18% of patients with unstable angina. Patients typically have a history of chest pain with normal or slightly elevated cardiac markers. The syndrome is characterized by specific ST-segment and T-wave changes that indicate a prein-farction state involving a critical proximal stenosis in the left anterior descending coronary artery. Identification and intervention of this syndrome before a myocardial infarction (MI) can reduce morbidity and mortality in these patients.

The characteristic precordial-lead electrocardiogram (ECG) changes include:
◆ no pathologic Q waves
◆ normal or minimally elevated ST segments
◆ T-wave changes:

    The most common T-wave change (shown here) is a deep symmetrical inversion.

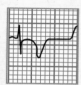 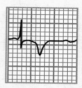

A less common T-wave change is a biphasic pattern (shown here).

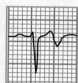 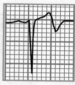

    Typically, ECG changes in Wellens syndrome involve leads V_2 and V_3; however, occasion-ally all precordial leads V_1 through V_6 may be involved. These characteristic changes fre-quently occur when the patient isn't experiencing chest pain. Early identification of Wellens syndrome and treatment of coronary artery stenosis can prevent an acute MI.

    Some patients experience a delay between the onset of pain and the appearance of certain ECG changes. Shown here are 12-lead ECGs for a patient with Wellens syndrome. The first tracing was recorded while the patient was experiencing chest pain. Yet, leads V_1, V_2, and V_3 show only slight T-wave changes (slight T-wave inversion at the end of the T wave). However, in the second tracing, which was taken 12 hours later when the patient was no longer experiencing pain, leads V_2 through V_6 show deeply inverted, symmetrical T waves and ST-segment abnormalities typical of Wellens syndrome.

(continued)

MI

● The initial step in assessing a pa-tient who's complaining of chest pain or other ischemic symptoms is to ob-tain a 12-lead ECG. This should be done within 10 minutes after the pa-tient has been seen by a practitioner.

It's a crucial component in determin-ing if MI is present. Interpretation of the ECG is the next step in identifying an ACS. The findings will direct the patient's treatment plan. (See *Stages of myocardial ischemia, injury, and infarct,* page 159.)

ECG during anginal pain

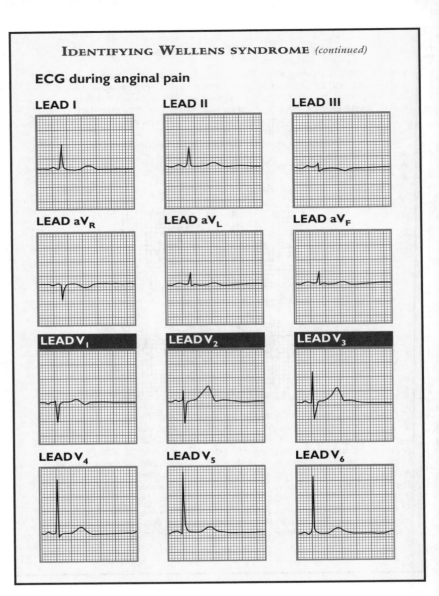

LEAD I	LEAD II	LEAD III

LEAD aV_R	LEAD aV_L	LEAD aV_F

LEAD V_1	LEAD V_2	LEAD V_3

LEAD V_4	LEAD V_5	LEAD V_6

● Patients should be classified as having ST-segment elevation or new left bundle-branch block (LBBB), ST-segment depression or dynamic T-wave inversion, or nondiagnostic or normal ECG.

ST-segment elevation or new LBBB
● Patients with an ST-segment elevation greater than or equal to 2 mm in two or more continuous leads or with new LBBB need to be treated for acute MI.

ECG after cessation of anginal pain

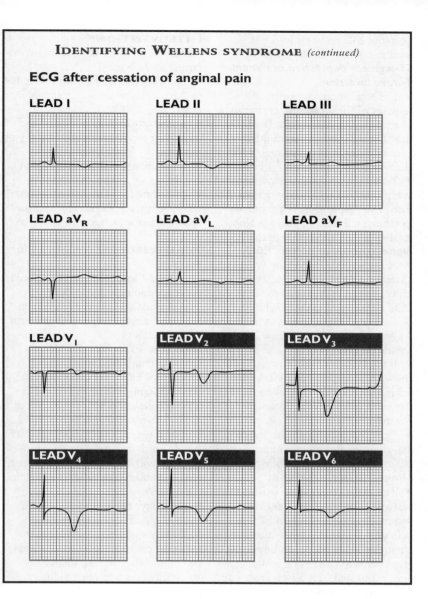

LEAD I LEAD II LEAD III
LEAD aV$_R$ LEAD aV$_L$ LEAD aV$_F$
LEAD V$_1$ LEAD V$_2$ LEAD V$_3$
LEAD V$_4$ LEAD V$_5$ LEAD V$_6$

● More than 90% of patients with this presentation will develop new pathologic Q waves and have positive cardiac markers in the blood.

● Repeating the ECG may be helpful for patients who present with peaked T waves.

● Patients with ST depression in leads V$_1$ and V$_2$ and with persistent symptoms may be evaluated for a posterior MI. Posterior-lead ECG is used to confirm the diagnosis.

ST-segment depression or dynamic T-wave inversion

- Ischemia should be suspected with findings of ST depression greater than or equal to 0.5 mm, marked symmetrical T-wave inversion in multiple precordial leads, and dynamic ST-T changes with pain.
- Patients who display persistent symptoms and recurrent ischemia, diffuse or widespread ECG abnormalities, heart failure, and positive blood markers are considered high risk.

Nondiagnostic or normal ECG

- A normal ECG won't show any ST changes or arrhythmias. However, at times, despite ischemia, a patient's ECG may appear normal, without ST or T wave changes. In this case, and if symptoms persist, repeat ECGs should be done.
- If the ECG is nondiagnostic, it may show an ST depression of less than 0.5 mm or a T-wave inversion or flattening in leads with dominant R waves.
- Continue assessment of myocardial changes through use of serial ECGs, ST-segment monitoring, and cardiac markers in the blood.
- The patient with acute pericarditis will also present with ST-segment elevation. Review the 12-lead ECG to help you determine if the patient is having an acute MI or has developed acute pericarditis. The patient with pericarditis will have ST-segment and T-wave changes in several leads; however, in acute MI the changes will be seen in the leads reflecting the area of infarction. (See *Comparing MI with acute pericarditis,* page 160, and *Identifying pericarditis*, page 161.)

INTERVENTIONS

Treatment goals for the patient experiencing an ACS include:

- reducing the amount of myocardial necrosis in those with ongoing infarction
- decreasing cardiac workload and increasing oxygen supply to the myocardium
- preventing major adverse cardiac events
- providing for rapid defibrillation when ventricular fibrillation or pulseless ventricular tachycardia is present.

Initial treatment measures for ACS

Obtain a 12-lead ECG and additional posterior and right precordial leads as necessary, and cardiac markers in the blood as ordered, to help confirm the diagnosis of acute MI. Cardiac biomarkers in the blood (especially troponin I and creatine kinase-myocardial band) are used to distinguish unstable angina and non–ST-segment elevation MI. (See *Release of cardiac enzymes and proteins,* page 162.)

Use the mnemonic MONA, which stands for morphine, oxygen, nitroglycerin, and aspirin, to start treatment for any patient experiencing ischemic chest pain or suspected ACS.

- Give oxygen to increase oxygenation of blood.
- Give non-enteric, coated aspirin to inhibit platelet aggregation, unless contraindicated. If the patient has an aspirin allergy, give clopidogrel (Plavix).
- Give nitroglycerin sublingually to dilate coronary blood vessels (unless systolic blood pressure is less than 110 mm Hg or heart rate is less than 50 beats/ minute or greater than 100 beats/ minute).

STAGES OF MYOCARDIAL ISCHEMIA, INJURY, AND INFARCT

Three stages occur when there's occlusion of a vessel: ischemia, injury, and infarct.

ISCHEMIA

Ischemia is the first stage; it indicates that blood flow and oxygen demand are out of balance. It can be resolved by improving flow or reducing oxygen needs. Electrocardiogram (ECG) changes indicate ST-segment depression or T-wave changes.

INJURY

The second stage, injury, occurs when the ischemia is prolonged enough to damage the area of the heart. ECG changes typically reveal ST-segment elevation (usually in two or more leads).

INFARCT

Infarct is the third stage and occurs with actual death of myocardial cells. Scar tissue eventually replaces the dead tissue, and the damage caused is irreversible.

In the earliest stage of a myocardial infarction (MI), peaked T waves may be seen on the ECG. Within hours, the T waves become inverted and ST-segment elevation occurs in the leads facing the area of damage.

The last change to occur in the evolution of an MI is the development of a pathologic Q wave, which is the only permanent ECG evidence of myocardial necrosis. Q waves are considered pathologic when they appear greater than or equal to 0.04 second wide and their height is greater than 25% of the R-wave height in that lead. Pathologic Q waves develop in more than 90% of patients with ST-segment elevation MI. Approximately 25% of patients with non–ST-segment elevation MI will develop pathologic Q waves and the remaining patients will have a non–Q-wave MI.

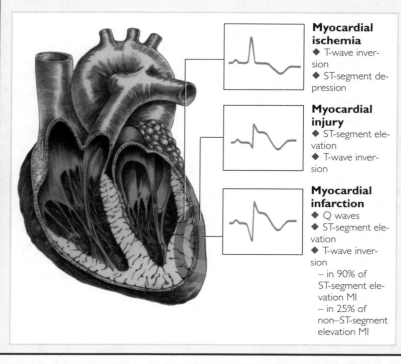

Myocardial ischemia
◆ T-wave inversion
◆ ST-segment depression

Myocardial injury
◆ ST-segment elevation
◆ T-wave inversion

Myocardial infarction
◆ Q waves
◆ ST-segment elevation
◆ T-wave inversion
  – in 90% of ST-segment elevation MI
  – in 25% of non–ST-segment elevation MI

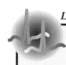

COMPARING MI WITH
ACUTE PERICARDITIS

Myocardial infarction (MI) and acute pericarditis cause ST-segment elevation on an electro-cardiogram (ECG). However, the ST segment and T wave (shaded areas) on an MI wave-form are quite different from those on the pericarditis waveform.

In addition, because pericarditis involves the surrounding pericardium, several leads will show ST-segment and T-wave changes (typically leads I, II, aV$_F$, and V$_4$ through V$_6$). In MI, though, only those leads reflecting the area of infarction will show the characteristic changes.

These rhythm strips demonstrate the ECG variations between MI and acute pericarditis.

MI

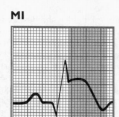

Acute pericarditis

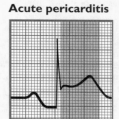

- Give morphine to relieve persistent pain or treat pulmonary edema.

For the patient with unstable angina and non–ST-segment elevation MI, treatment includes the above initial measures as well as:
- giving beta-adrenergic blockers to reduce the heart's workload and oxygen demands
- giving heparin and glycoprotein IIb/IIIa inhibitors to minimize platelet aggregation and danger of coronary occlusion with high-risk patients (patients with planned cardiac catheterization and positive troponin)
- administering I.V. nitroglycerin to reduce myocardial workload by promoting vasodilation of the peripheral blood vessel, relieving chest pain (unless systolic blood pressure is less than 110 mm Hg or heart rate is less than 50 beats/minute or greater than 100 beats/minute)

- if the patient has an arrhythmia, preparing for use of antiarrhythmics, transcutaneous pacing patches (or transvenous pacemaker), or defibrillation
- performing percutaneous transluminal coronary angioplasty (PTCA) or coronary artery bypass graft (CABG) surgery for obstructive lesions
- giving antilipemic drugs to reduce elevated cholesterol or triglyceride levels in the blood.

For the patient with ST-segment elevation MI, treatment includes the above initial measures as well as:
- providing thrombolytic therapy (unless contraindicated) within 12 hours of onset of symptoms to restore vessel patency and minimize necrosis in ST-segment elevation MI
- administering heparin to promote patency in affected coronary artery

IDENTIFYING PERICARDITIS

Pericarditis is an inflammation of the pericardium—the fibroserous sac that envelops the heart. Pericarditis can be either acute or chronic. The acute form may be fibrinous or effusive, with purulent, serous, or hemorrhagic exudate. Chronic constrictive pericarditis causes dense fibrous thickening of the pericardium. Possible causes of pericarditis include:
◆ viral, bacterial, or fungal disorders
◆ rheumatic fever
◆ autoimmune disorders
◆ complications of cardiac injury (myocardial infarction, cardiotomy).

Regardless of the form, pericarditis can cause cardiac tamponade if fluid accumulates too quickly. It also can cause heart failure if constriction occurs.

Electrocardiogram changes in acute pericarditis evolve through two stages:
◆ **Stage 1**—Diffuse ST-segment elevations of 1 to 2 mm in most limb leads and most precordial leads reflect the inflammatory process. Upright T waves are present in most leads. The ST-segment and T-wave changes are typically seen in leads I, II, III, aV_L, aV_F, and V_2 through V_6.
◆ **Stage 2**—As pericarditis resolves, the ST-segment elevation and accompanying T-wave inversion resolves in most leads.

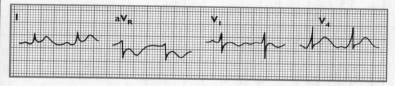

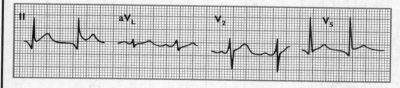

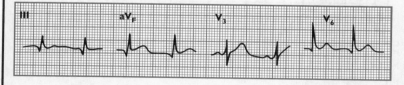

● giving beta-adrenergic blockers to reduce myocardial workload
● giving glycoprotein IIb/IIIa inhibitors to reduce platelet aggregation
● if the patient has an arrhythmia, preparing for use of antiarrhythmics, transcutaneous pacing patches (or transvenous pacemaker), or defibrillation
● giving angiotensin-converting enzyme inhibitors to reduce afterload and preload and prevent remodeling
● performing interventional procedures, such as PTCA, stent placement,

RELEASE OF CARDIAC ENZYMES AND PROTEINS

Because they're released by damaged tissue, serum proteins and isoenzymes (catalytic proteins that vary in concentration in specific organs) can help identify the compromised organ and assess the extent of damage. After acute myocardial infarction, cardiac enzymes and proteins rise and fall in a characteristic pattern, as shown in the graph below.

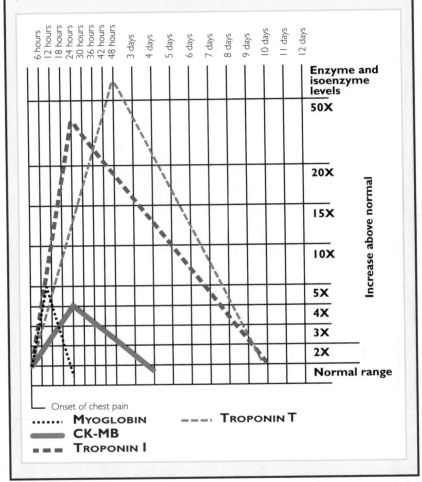

or surgical procedures, such as CABG, which may open blocked or narrowed arteries.

LOCATIONS OF MI

The location of the MI is a critical factor in determining the most appropriate treatment and predicting probable

LOCATING MYOCARDIAL DAMAGE

After you've noted characteristic electrocardiogram lead changes in an acute myocardial infarction, use this table to identify the areas of damage. Match the lead changes (ST elevation, abnormal Q waves) in the second column with the affected wall in the first column and the artery involved in the third column. The fourth column shows reciprocal lead changes.

WALL AFFECTED	LEADS	ARTERY INVOLVED	RECIPROCAL LEAD CHANGES
Anterior	V_2, V_3, V_4	Left coronary artery, left anterior descending (LAD) artery	II, III, aV_F
Anterolateral	I, aV_L, V_2, V_3, V_4, V_5, V_6	LAD artery and diagonal branches, circumflex and marginal branches	II, III, aV_F
Anteroseptal	V_1, V_2, V_3, V_4	LAD artery	None
Inferior	II, III, aV_F	Right coronary artery (RCA)	I, aV_L
Lateral	I, aV_L, V_5, V_6	Circumflex branch of left coronary artery	II, III, aV_F
Posterior	V_8, V_9	RCA or circumflex	V_1, V_2, V_3, V_4 (R greater than S in V_1 and V_2, ST-segment depression, elevated T wave)
Right ventricular	V_{4R}, V_{5R}, V_{6R}	RCA	None

complications. Characteristic ECG changes that occur with each type of MI are localized to the leads overlying the infarction site. (See *Locating myocardial damage.*) This section takes a look at characteristic ECG changes that occur with different types of MIs.

Anterior wall MI

The left anterior descending artery supplies blood to the anterior portion of the left ventricle, ventricular septum, and portions of the right and left bundle-branch systems.

When the left anterior descending artery becomes occluded, an anterior wall MI occurs. (See *Identifying an anterior wall MI,* page 164.) Complications include second-degree atrioventricular blocks, bundle-branch blocks, ventric-

ular irritability, and left-sided heart failure.

An anterior wall MI causes characteristic ECG changes in leads V_2 to V_4. The precordial leads show poor R-wave progression because the left ventricle can't depolarize normally. ST-segment elevation and T-wave inversion are also present.

The reciprocal leads for the anterior wall are the inferior leads II, III, and aV_F. They initially show tall R waves and depressed ST segments.

Septal wall MI

The patient with a septal wall MI is at increased risk for developing a ventricular septal defect. ECG changes are present in leads V_1 and V_2. In those leads, the R wave disappears, the ST

IDENTIFYING AN ANTERIOR WALL MI

This 12-lead electrocardiogram shows typical characteristics of an anterior wall myocardial infarction (MI). Note that the R waves don't progress through the precordial leads. Also note the ST-segment elevation in leads V_2 and V_3. As expected, the reciprocal leads II, III, and aV_F show slight ST-segment depression. Axis is normal at +60 degrees.

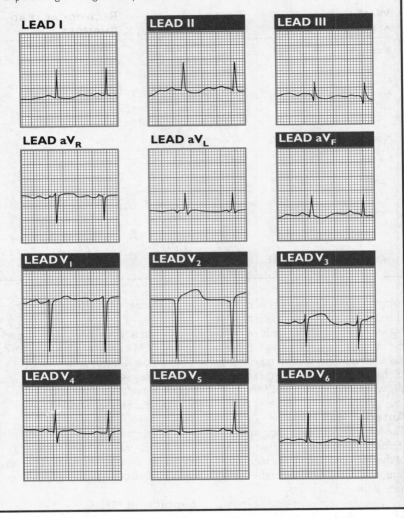

segment rises, and the T wave inverts. Because the left anterior descending artery also supplies blood to the ven- tricular septum, a septal wall MI typically accompanies an anterior wall MI.

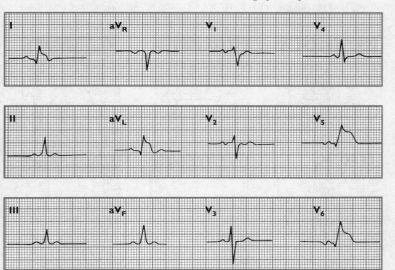

IDENTIFYING A LATERAL WALL MI

This 12-lead electrocardiogram shows typical characteristics of a lateral wall myocardial infarction (MI). Note the ST-segment elevation in leads I, aV$_L$, V$_5$, and V$_6$.

Lateral wall MI

A lateral wall MI is usually caused by a blockage in the left circumflex artery and shows characteristic changes in the left lateral leads I, aV$_L$, V$_5$, and V$_6$. The reciprocal leads for a lateral wall infarction are leads II, III, and aV$_F$. (See *Identifying a lateral wall MI.*)

A lateral wall MI typically causes premature ventricular contractions (PVCs) and varying degrees of heart block. It may accompany an anterior or inferior wall MI.

Inferior wall MI

An inferior wall MI is usually caused by occlusion of the right coronary artery and produces characteristic ECG changes in the inferior leads II, III, and aV$_F$ and reciprocal changes in the lateral leads I and aV$_L$. (See *Identifying an inferior wall MI*, page 166.) It's also called a *diaphragmatic MI* because the inferior wall of the heart lies over the diaphragm.

Patients with inferior wall MI are at risk for developing sinus bradycardia, sinus arrest, heart block, and PVCs. This type of MI occurs alone or with a lateral wall, posterior wall, or right ventricular MI.

Posterior wall MI

A posterior wall MI is caused by occlusion of the right coronary artery or the left circumflex arteries. It produces reciprocal changes in leads V$_1$ to V$_4$.

ECG changes for a posterior wall MI include tall R waves, ST-segment

IDENTIFYING AN INFERIOR WALL MI

This 12-lead electrocardiogram (ECG) shows the characteristic changes of an inferior wall myocardial infarction (MI). In leads II, III, and aV_F, note the T-wave inversion, ST-segment elevation, and pathologic Q waves. In leads I and aV_L, note the slight ST-segment depression—a reciprocal change. This ECG shows left axis deviation at -60 degrees.

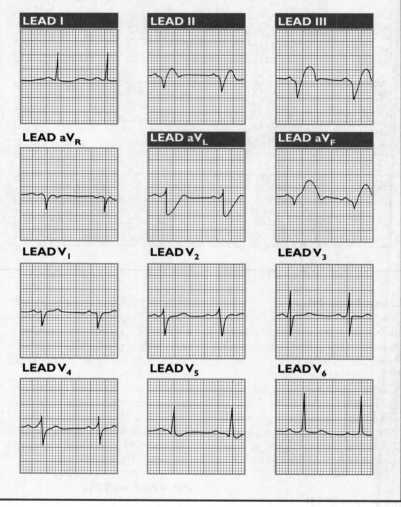

depression, and upright T waves. Posterior infarctions may accompany inferior infarctions. Data about the posterior wall and pathologic Q waves that might occur can be obtained from

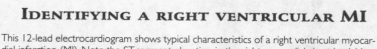

IDENTIFYING A RIGHT VENTRICULAR MI

This 12-lead electrocardiogram shows typical characteristics of a right ventricular myocardial infarction (MI). Note the ST-segment elevation in the right precordial chest leads V_{4R}, V_{5R}, and V_{6R}. Pathologic Q waves would also appear in leads V_{4R}, V_{5R}, and V_{6R}.

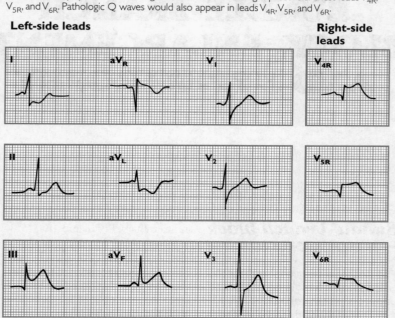

Left-side leads

Right-side leads

leads V_8 and V_9, using a posterior ECG.

Right ventricular MI

A right ventricular MI usually follows occlusion of the right coronary artery. This type of MI rarely occurs alone. In 40% of patients, a right ventricular MI accompanies an inferior wall MI. (See *Identifying a right ventricular MI*.)

A right ventricular MI can lead to right ventricular failure. The classic changes are ST-segment elevation, pathologic Q waves, and inverted T waves in the right precordial leads V_{2R} to V_{6R}. Identifying a right ventricular MI is difficult without informa-

tion from the right precordial leads. If these leads aren't available, you can observe leads II, III, and aV_F or watch leads V_1 and V_2 for ST-segment elevation.

13

BUNDLE-BRANCH BLOCK, ENLARGEMENT, AND HYPERTROPHY

Bundle-branch block

With *bundle-branch block* (BBB), either the left or right bundle branch fails to conduct impulses normally. A BBB that occurs toward the distal end of the left bundle, in the posterior or anterior fasciculus, is called a *fascicular block* or *hemiblock*. Some blocks require treatment with a temporary pacemaker. Others are monitored only to detect whether they progress to a more complex block.

In BBB, the impulse travels down the unaffected bundle branch and then from one myocardial cell to the next to depolarize the ventricle. Because this cell-to-cell conduction progresses much more slowly than it does along the specialized cells of the conduction system, ventricular depolarization is prolonged.

Prolonged ventricular depolarization means that the QRS complex widens. The normal QRS duration is 0.06 to 0.10 second. A QRS complex

duration more than 0.12 second may indicate that a BBB is present.

After identifying BBB, examine lead V_1 and lead V_6 on the 12-lead electrocardiogram (ECG). You'll use these leads to determine whether the block is in the right or left bundle branch.

Both temporary and permanent heart blocks may be associated with acute myocardial infarction (MI). An acute MI, in fact, is the primary cause of heart blocks. Other causes include atherosclerosis, valvular disease, ventricular hypertrophy, infective cardiac disease, congenital abnormalities, and cardiac drugs that alter the refractory period of interventricular conduction.

The different types of heart block stem from different causes and have different implications for the patient. The different types include:
- right bundle-branch block (RBBB)
- left bundle-branch block (LBBB)
- left anterior fascicular block (LAFB) (also called *anterior hemiblock*)
- left posterior fascicular block (LPFB) (also called *posterior hemiblock*)

- trifascicular block.

With BBB, you may see an extra notch in the R wave, called *R prime* (R'), or an extra notch in the S wave, called *S prime* (S'). And, of course, each type of BBB produces distinctive changes on a 12-lead ECG.

RIGHT BUNDLE-BRANCH BLOCK

When RBBB occurs, the impulse still activates the interventricular septum from left to right, but then the impulse activates the left ventricle before activating the right ventricle. (See *Understanding RBBB,* page 170.)

Causes

Causes of RBBB include:
- acute heart failure
- anterior wall MI,
- atrial septal defect
- cardiac catheterization of the right heart
- congenital anomalies
- coronary artery disease (CAD)
- hypokalemia
- pulmonary embolism
- rheumatic heart disease
- right ventricular hypertrophy
- valvular heart disease.

It also may occur without cardiac disease. If it develops as the heart rate increases, it's called *rate-related RBBB.*

ECG characteristics

Rhythm: Atrial and ventricular rhythms regular
Rate: Atrial and ventricular rates within normal limits
P wave: May be normal in size and configuration
PR interval: Within normal limits
QRS complex: Duration appearing at least 0.12 second in complete block and 0.10 and 0.12 second in incomplete block. (In lead V_1, the QRS complex is wide and can appear in one of several patterns: an rSR' complex with a wide S and R' wave; an rSR' complex with a wide R wave; and a wide R wave with an M-shaped pattern. The complex is mainly positive, with the R wave occurring late. In leads I, aV_L, and V_6, a broad S wave greater than 0.12 second can be seen, and has a different configuration, sometimes resembling rabbit ears or the letter "M." (See *Identifying RBBB,* page 171.)
T wave: In most leads, deflection appearing opposite that of the QRS deflection
QT interval: May be prolonged or within normal limits
Other: In precordial leads, triphasic complexes occurring because the right ventricle continues to depolarize after the left ventricle depolarizes, thereby producing a third phase of ventricular stimulation

Signs and symptoms

Typically there are no signs or symptoms of RBBB. Auscultation may reveal a fixed splitting of the second heart sound (S_2).

Interventions

Treatment aims to correct the underlying problem. A pacemaker may be needed if RBBB occurs with an acute anteroseptal MI, especially if there's a preexisting left anterior or posterior fascicular block.

LEFT BUNDLE-BRANCH BLOCK

In LBBB, conduction through the left ventricle is impaired. A block may be located on the main bundle, or blocks may be located on both the anterior and posterior fascicles.

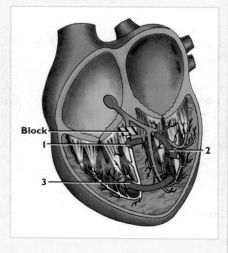
With LBBB, ventricular activation occurs in this order: First, the right ventricle is activated by the right bundle branch. Then the interventricular septum is activated abnormally in a right-to-left direction. Finally, the left ventricle is activated. (See *Understanding LBBB,* page 172.)

Causes

When LBBB is discovered on a routine ECG, the patient may have hypertensive ischemic disease, primary heart disease, or no serious heart disease at all.

The most common causes of LBBB are:
- hypertensive cardiovascular disease
- severe CAD
- valvular disease
  Other causes include:
- cardiomyopathy
- congenital lesions
- Lenègre's disease
- Lev's disease
- rheumatic disease.

ECG characteristics

Rhythm: Atrial and ventricular rhythms regular, depending on the underlying rhythm

Rate: Atrial and ventricular rates usually within normal limits

P wave: Normal in size and configuration

PR interval: Within normal limits

QRS complex: Duration varying from 0.10 and 0.12 second in incomplete LBBB; appearing at least 0.12 second in complete block; lead V_1 showing a wide, largely negative rS complex or entirely negative QS complex; leads I, AV_L, and V_6 showing a wide, tall R wave without a Q or S wave (see *Identifying LBBB,* page 173)

T wave: In most leads, deflection appearing opposite that of the QRS deflection

IDENTIFYING RBBB

This 12-lead electrocardiogram shows the characteristic changes of right bundle-branch block (RBBB). In lead V_1, note the rsR' pattern and T-wave inversion. In lead V_6, see the widened S wave and the upright T wave. Also note the prolonged QRS complexes.

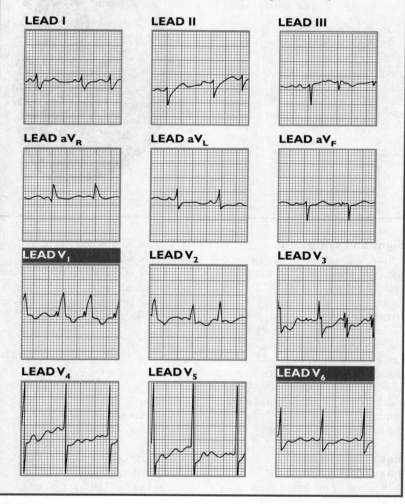

QT interval: May be prolonged or within normal limits
Other: Magnitude of changes paralleling the magnitude of the QRS complex aberration; axis may be normal or showing left axis deviation; delayed intrinsicoid deflection over the left ventricle (lead V_6)

UNDERSTANDING LBBB

In left bundle-branch block (LBBB), the impulse first travels down the right bundle branch (arrow 1). Then the impulse activates the interventricular septum from right to left (arrow 2), the opposite of normal activation. Finally, the impulse activates the left ventricle (arrow 3).

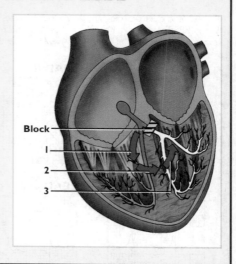

Signs and symptoms

Typically there are no signs or symptoms of LBBB. Auscultation may reveal a fixed splitting of S_2.

Interventions

Treatment aims to correct the underlying problem. For the patient who's had an acute MI, a pacemaker may be inserted because of the increased risk of complete atrioventricular (AV) block. A ventricular pacemaker may improve symptoms of heart failure in the patient with a large LBBB.

LEFT ANTERIOR FASCICULAR BLOCK

A blockage of the left anterior fascicle causes the left ventricle to be activated by the left posterior fascicle only. Impulses from this fascicle depolarize the inferior and posterior walls of the left ventricle. The right ventricle is depolarized by the right bundle branch at the same time. This depolarization ini-

tially causes the impulse to be aimed downward and to the right. After reaching the Purkinje network, the impulse activates the anterior, lateral, and upper left ventricular walls. (See *Understanding LAFB,* page 174.)

Causes

LAFB (also called *left anterior hemiblock*) can occur with an inferior wall MI, but it's more common with an acute anterior wall MI.

Other causes include:
- aortic valve disease
- CAD
- cardiomyopathies
- degenerative conduction disorders such as Lev's or Lenègre's disease.
- hyperkalemia
- hypertension
- myocarditis
- normal aging.

IDENTIFYING LBBB

This 12-lead electrocardiogram shows characteristic changes of a left bundle-branch block (LBBB). All leads have prolonged QRS complexes. In lead V_1, note the QS wave pattern. In lead V_6, you'll see the wide and tall R wave and T-wave inversion. The elevated ST segments and upright T waves in leads V_1 to V_4 are also common in LBBB.

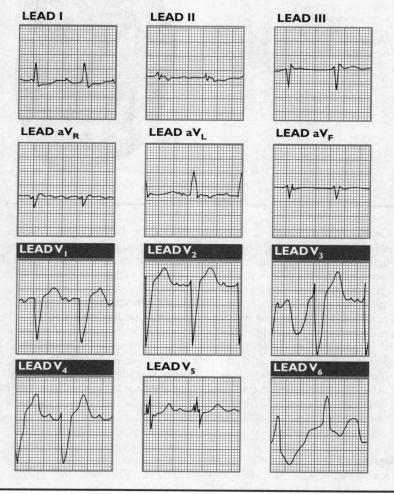

LEAD I LEAD II LEAD III

LEAD aV_R LEAD aV_L LEAD aV_F

LEAD V_1 LEAD V_2 LEAD V_3

LEAD V_4 LEAD V_5 LEAD V_6

ECG characteristics

Rhythm: Atrial and ventricular rhythms regular, depending on the underlying rhythm

Rate: Atrial and ventricular rates usually within normal limits

P wave: Normal in size and configuration

Understanding LAFB

In left anterior fascicular block (LAFB), the left ventricle is activated by the left posterior fascicle only (arrow 1), causing the impulse to be aimed downward and to the right initially. The right ventricle is depolarized by the right bundle branch at the same time (arrow 2). After the impulse reaches the Purkinje network, the impulse activates the anterior, lateral, and upper left ventricular walls (arrow 3).

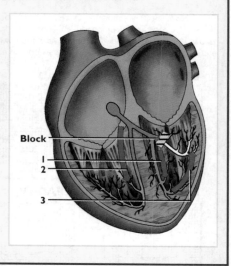

Block

1
2

3

PR interval: Within normal limits
QRS complex: Duration appearing prolonged, but may fall within normal limits—0.10 second or less; small Q wave appearing in lead I and a small R wave in lead III; a deep S wave in lead II; a deeper S wave in lead III; and an rS pattern in leads II and III (see *Identifying LAFB*)
QT interval: May be prolonged or within normal limits
T wave: May be inverted in leads I and aV_L and upright in leads II, III, and aV_F
Other: Left axis deviation usually −45 degrees or greater

Signs and symptoms
There are usually no signs and symptoms associated with LAFB.

Interventions
Treatment usually isn't necessary for LAFB. If the fascicular block occurs with an acute anteroseptal MI, a pacemaker may be needed, especially if the patient also has RBBB. If the patient has had an MI, monitor the modified chest lead (MCL_1) or V_1, and also watch for the development of RBBB.

Left posterior fascicular block
With LPFB, the left anterior fascicle depolarizes the anterior and lateral walls of the left ventricle first. The right ventricle is depolarized by the right bundle branch at the same time. The impulse then crosses the Purkinje network and activates the inferior and posterior walls of the left ventricle. The impulse first moves to the left and anteriorly, then to the right and inferiorly. (See *Understanding LPFB*, page 176.)

Causes
LPFB (also called *left posterior hemiblock*) usually occurs with an acute MI, CAD, or ischemia.

IDENTIFYING LAFB

This 12-lead electrocardiogram shows characteristic changes of left anterior fascicular block (LAFB). Occurring in the anterosuperior fascicle of the left bundle branch, LAFB causes ventricular activation through the posteroinferior fascicle. As a result, left axis deviation takes place. Although less serious than a left posterior fascicular block, LAFB frequently occurs with right bundle-branch block or anterior myocardial infarction.

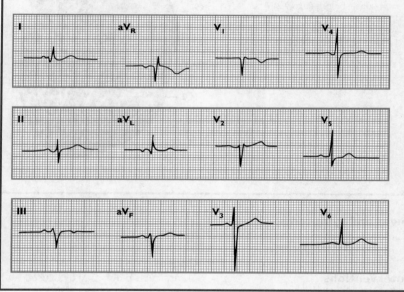

Other causes include:
- aging
- cardiomyopathy
- conduction system sclerosis
- hyperkalemia
- hypertension.

ECG characteristics

Rhythm: Atrial and ventricular rhythms regular, depending on the underlying rhythm

Rate: Atrial and ventricular rates usually within normal limits

P wave: Normal in size and configuration

PR interval: Within normal limits

QRS complex: Duration appearing prolonged, but may fall within normal limits—0.10 second or less; small Q wave appearing in leads III, a small R wave in lead I, and a deep S wave in lead I; large QRS complex in the precordial leads resulting from increased voltage (see *Identifying LPFB,* page 177)

T wave: May be inverted in leads I and aV$_L$ and upright in leads II, III, and aV$_F$

QT interval: May be prolonged or within normal limits

Other: Mean QRS axis usually at least +120 degrees (right axis deviation) reflected by a negative lead I and a positive lead aV$_F$

UNDERSTANDING LPFB

In left posterior fascicular block (LPFB), the left anterior fascicle depolarizes the anterolateral wall of the left ventricle (arrow I); at the same time, the right ventricle will be depolarized by the right bundle branch (arrow 2). After the impulse reaches the Purkinje network, it activates the inferoposterior wall of the left ventricle (arrow 3).

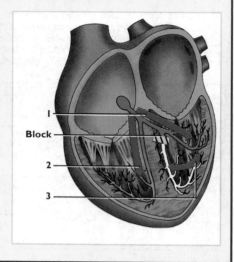

Signs and symptoms
There are usually no signs and symptoms associated with LPFB.

Interventions
Treatment usually isn't necessary for LPFB. If the fascicular block occurs with an acute anteroseptal MI, a pacemaker may be needed, especially if the patient has RBBB. If the patient has had an MI, monitor MCL_1 or V_1, and watch for the development of RBBB. If complete heart block results from RBBB with LPFB, treatment attempts to support and maintain a stable ventricular rhythm.

TRIFASCICULAR BLOCK
In trifascicular block, the intraventricular conduction abnormality involves the right bundle branch and also the anterior and posterior fascicles of the left bundle branch—this may be a form of complete heart block.

Causes
Trifascicular block may be caused by an MI, cardiac disease, or medications.

ECG characteristics
Trifascicular block exists when first-degree AV block is present in combination with LBBB involving both fascicles of the left bundle. Trifascicular block is also present when there is a first-degree AV block, along with RBBB and LAFB or LPFB.

Signs and symptoms
Depending on the heart rate, the patient may experience syncope, dizziness, chest pain, or shortness of breath, or there may not be any signs or symptoms.

IDENTIFYING LPFB

This 12-lead electrocardiogram shows characteristic changes of left posterior fascicular block (LPFB). Occurring in the posteroinferior fascicle of the left bundle branch, LPFB causes ventricular activation through the anterosuperior fascicle. As a result, right axis deviation takes place. This arrhythmia is more serious than a left anterior fascicular block because it's associated with a larger lesion blocking the broad posterior fascicle. When a right bundle-branch block occurs with LPFB, the likelihood of complete heart block is increased.

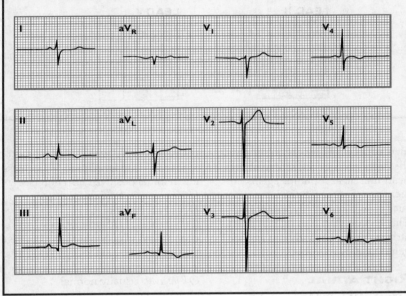

Interventions

Treatment aims to correct the underlying condition. Monitor the block to determine whether it becomes more extensive. It's recommended to have a transcutaneous pacemaker on standby in case the patient develops complete heart block.

When RBBB occurs after an anterior wall MI, some physicians insert a temporary transvenous pacemaker as a preventive measure. A permanent pacemaker may be inserted if the condition is chronic.

Enlargement and hypertrophy

The atria and ventricles can enlarge because of an increase in pressure or volume. The atria, which are thin-walled, usually dilate in response to an increase in pressure and volume. The ventricles, which are thick-walled, dilate with increased volume and hypertrophy with increased pressure.

Hypertrophy is an increase in the size of a cell or organ because of an

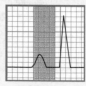
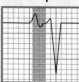
increase in workload. Hypertrophy in the heart refers to thickening of the heart muscle as it pumps against increasing resistance in the heart vessels, such as occurs with hypertension. This section discusses right and left atrial enlargement and right and left ventricular hypertrophy.

RIGHT ATRIAL ENLARGEMENT

Right atrial enlargement affects the P wave because of the initial part of the P wave occurring from right atrial depolarization.

Causes

Causes of right atrial enlargement include:
- chronic obstructive lung disease
- pulmonary emboli
- tricuspid insufficiency
- tricuspid stenosis.

ECG characteristics

Rhythm: Atrial and ventricular rhythms normal
Rate: Atrial and ventricular rates normal

P wave: Peaked P wave in lead II greater than 2.5 mm amplitude; V_1 increasing in initial positive deflection (see *Identifying right atrial enlargement*)
PR interval: Normal
QRS complex: QRS voltage in V_1 appearing less than 5 mm above baseline
ST segment: Normal
T wave: Normal
QT interval: Usually normal
Other: None

Signs and symptoms

Signs and symptoms are related to the underlying disorder.

Interventions

Treatment focuses on management of the underlying disorder, such as hypertension.

LEFT ATRIAL ENLARGEMENT

Left atrial enlargement causes delay in the electrical activity of the left atrium, resulting in a change in the shape of the P wave.

The waveforms here show key electrocardiogram changes that occur in selected leads with the presence of left atrial enlargement.

In lead II, the P wave is notched (see shaded area). In lead V_1, you'll see a biphasic P wave with an initial positive deflection followed by a prominent negative deflection in the terminal portion of the wave (see shaded area). In both leads, the P wave duration is increased.

LEAD II

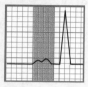

LEAD V₁

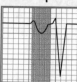

Causes

Left atrial enlargement may occur with mitral valve stenosis or mitral insufficiency. It also commonly occurs with any cause of left ventricular enlargement.

ECG characteristics

Rhythm: Atrial and ventricular rhythms normal
Rate: Atrial and ventricular rates normal
P wave: P wave duration of 0.11 msec or longer; notching of the P wave with the peaks being more than 1 mm apart and prominence of the terminal portion of the P wave, or prominent negativity of the terminal portion of the P wave in lead V_1 (see *Identifying left atrial enlargement*)
PR interval: Normal
QRS complex: Normal
ST segment: Normal
T wave: Normal
QT interval: Usually normal

Signs and symptoms

Signs and symptoms are related to the underlying disorder.

Interventions

Treatment focuses on management of the underlying disorder such as hypertension.

RIGHT VENTRICULAR HYPERTROPHY

In *right ventricular hypertrophy* (RVH), the right ventricular wall thickens. RVH usually results from conditions that cause chronic increases in pressures within the ventricle.

Causes

Causes of RVH include:
- primary pulmonary hypertension
- pulmonary valve stenosis
- right ventricle outflow obstruction (may occur with pulmonary disease)
- tetralogy of Fallot
- ventricular septal defect.

ECG characteristics

Rhythm: Atrial and ventricular rhythms normal
Rate: Atrial and ventricular rates normal

IDENTIFYING RVH

The waveforms here show key electrocardiogram changes that occur in selected leads with the presences of right ventricular hypertrophy (RVH).

Normally, the R wave would progressively increase from V_1 to V_6. In RVH, the R wave gets progressively smaller from V_1 to V_6. In lead V_1, you'll note a tall R wave (see shaded area). In lead V_6, the S wave is deepened (see shaded area) and the amplitude of the S wave is equal to or greater than that of the R wave (see arrows).

LEAD V₁

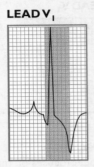

LEAD V₆

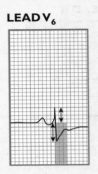

P wave: May be normal in size and configuration, or may reflect right atrial enlargement

PR interval: Normal

QRS complex: R wave getting progressively smaller from V_1 to V_6 (normally it would increase) and there's a deep S wave in V_5 or V_6; normal or slightly increased QRS duration (see *Identifying RVH*)

ST segment: Depression may occur

T wave: Inverted in V_1 and V_2

QT interval: Usually normal

Other: Right axis deviation may be present

Signs and symptoms

Signs and symptoms may be related to the underlying cause. With pulmonary hypertension and RVH, the patient may experience dizziness, shortness of breath, or syncope.

Interventions

Treatment focuses on management of the underlying disorder, such as pulmonary hypertension.

LEFT VENTRICULAR HYPERTROPHY

In *left ventricular hypertrophy* (LVH), the left ventricular wall thickens. LVH usually results from conditions that cause chronic increases in pressure within the ventricle.

Causes

Causes of LVH include:
● aortic stenosis or insufficiency
● cardiomyopathy
● mitral insufficiency
● systemic hypertension (most common cause).

LVH may lead to left-sided heart failure, which subsequently leads to increased left atrial pressure, pulmo-

IDENTIFYING LVH

Left ventricular hypertrophy (LVH) can lead to heart failure or myocardial infarction. The rhythm strips shown here illustrate key electrocardiogram changes of LVH as they occur in selected leads: a large S wave (shaded area below left) in V_1 and a large R wave (shaded area below right) in V_5. If the depth (in mm) of the S wave in V_1 added to the height (in mm) of the R wave in V_5 is greater than 35 mm, then LVH is present.

LEAD V_1   **LEAD V_6**

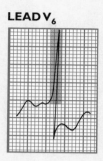

nary vascular congestion, and pulmonary arterial hypertension. LVH can decrease coronary artery perfusion, causing MI, or it can alter the papillary muscle, causing mitral insufficiency.

ECG characteristics

Rhythm: Atrial and ventricular rhythms normal
Rate: Atrial and ventricular rates normal
P wave: May be normal in size and configuration, or may reflect left atrial enlargement
PR interval: Normal
QRS complex: May be prolonged or widened with increased amplitude; increasing amplitude of R wave in leads I, aV_L, V_5, and V_6; S wave amplitude increasing in leads V_1 and V_2; LVH existing if depth of S wave in V_1 added to the height of R wave in V_5 appears greater than 35 mm (see *Identifying LVH*)

ST segment: Possibly depressed in the precordial leads when associated with T-wave inversion; this pattern known as LVH with strain
T wave: May be inverted in leads V_5 or V_6 depending on the degree of hypertrophy
QT interval: Usually normal
Other: Axis usually normal, but left axis deviation may be present

Signs and symptoms
Signs and symptoms are related to the underlying disorder.

Interventions
Treatment focuses on management of the underlying disorder such as hypertension.

PART 4

---◆---

Understanding the effects of treatment

14

PHARMACOLOGIC TREATMENTS FOR ARRHYTHMIAS

Almost half a million Americans die each year from cardiac arrhythmias; countless others experience symptoms that are severe enough to warrant lifestyle modifications. Along with other treatments, *cardiac drugs* can help alleviate symptoms, control heart rate and rhythm, and decrease preload and afterload, ultimately prolonging life.

This chapter reviews ECG changes that occur when patients take therapeutic doses of antiarrhythmics and digoxin. When drug levels are toxic, ECG changes are typically exaggerated.

Understanding antiarrhythmics

Antiarrhythmics affect the movement of ions across the cell membrane and alter the electrophysiology of the cardiac cell. These drugs are classified according to their effect on the cell's electrical activity (*action potential*) and their mechanism of action. Because the drugs can change the myocardial action potential, characteristic electrocardiogram (ECG) alterations can oc-

cur. (See *Antiarrhythmics and the action potential,* page 186.)

The classification system divides antiarrhythmics into four major classes based on their dominant mechanism of action: class I, class II, class III, and class IV. Class I antiarrhythmics are further divided into class IA, class IB, and class IC.

Certain antiarrhythmics can't be classified specifically into one group. For example, sotalol possesses characteristics of both class II and class III drugs. Other drugs, such as adenosine, atropine, digoxin, epinephrine, vasopressin, and magnesium, don't fit into the classification system at all. Despite its limitations, however, the classification system is helpful in understanding how antiarrhythmics prevent and treat arrhythmias.

DRUG DISTRIBUTION AND CLEARANCE

When you give an antiarrhythmic by infusion, blood levels will initially be high in well-perfused organs, such as the heart, liver, and kidneys.

Alert *Drug-induced arrhythmias are more likely to occur early in treatment when drug concentrations are higher.*

As the drug is distributed throughout the rest of the body, drug concen-

ANTIARRHYTHMICS AND THE ACTION POTENTIAL

Each class of antiarrhythmics acts on a different phase of the cardiac action potential to alter the heart's electrophysiology.

CLASS I DRUGS

Class I drugs are sodium channel blockers that reduce the influx of sodium ions into the cell during phase 0 of the action potential.

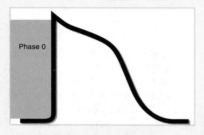

CLASS III DRUGS

Class III drugs are potassium channel blockers that prolong phase 3 of the action potential, thereby increasing repolarization and refractoriness.

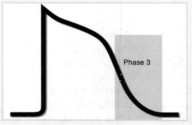

CLASS II DRUGS

Class II drugs inhibit adrenergic stimulation of cardiac tissue. They depress phase 4 spontaneous depolarization and slow sinoatrial node impulses.

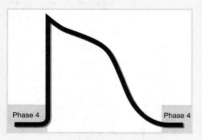

CLASS IV DRUGS

Class IV drugs inhibit calcium's slow influx into the cell during the action potential's plateau phase (phase 2). They depress phase 4 and lengthen phases 1 and 2.

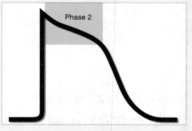

trations in these organs will diminish, along with the risk of toxicity and drug-induced arrhythmias.

Most antiarrhythmics are metabolized in the liver and excreted by the kidneys. As a result, altered blood flow to these organs can affect drug metabolism and clearance and increase the risk of toxicity. Alterations can also result from decreased cardiac output, compromised renal function, and concurrent administration of drugs that induce hepatic enzymes.

PROARRHYTHMIC EFFECTS

Antiarrhythmics can be *proarrhythmic;* that is, they cause or worsen arrhythmias. These arrhythmias may include sustained ventricular tachycardia, ventricular fibrillation, torsades de pointes, and ventricular standstill. Although the exact mechanisms that trigger proarrhythmias are unknown, certain factors may predispose the patient. Major risk factors include fluid and electrolyte imbalances and structural damage to the myocardium, particularly ischemic tissue injury.

When the patient experiences an electrolyte imbalance, changes in pH and circulating levels of catecholamines may increase the proarrhythmic effect of some antiarrhythmics. In the patient with myocardial ischemia, an antiarrhythmic may not only suppress abnormal rhythms that originate in diseased tissue but also may depress healthy tissue and prolong the action potential and delay ventricular repolarization.

When the patient is receiving an antiarrhythmic, be aware of these additional risk factors for proarrhythmias:

- a history of sustained ventricular tachycardia or ventricular fibrillation
- coronary artery disease or significant valvular disease
- severe left ventricular dysfunction
- electrolyte imbalance, particularly hypokalemia or hypomagnesemia
- history of long QT syndrome.

Class I antiarrhythmics

Class I antiarrhythmics block the influx of sodium into the cell during phase 0 of the action potential. Because phase 0 is also referred to as the *sodium channel* or *fast channel,* these drugs may also be called *sodium channel blockers* or *fast channel blockers.* Class I antiarrhythmics are frequently subdivided into three groups—A, B, and C—according to their interactions with cardiac sodium channels or the drug's effects on the duration of the action potential.

Class IA

Class IA antiarrhythmics include disopyramide, procainamide, and quinidine. These drugs lengthen the duration of the action potential, and their interaction with the sodium channels is classified as intermediate. As a result, conductivity is reduced and repolarization is prolonged. These drugs are used to treat supraventricular arrhythmias, such as paroxysmal supraventricular tachycardia, atrial flutter and atrial fibrillation, and ventricular arrhythmias such as premature ventricular contractions. Procainamide is also used to treat recurrent ventricular tachycardia and ventricular fibrillation.

ECG characteristics

Rhythm strip characteristics for a patient taking an antiarrhythmic vary according to the drug's classification. When a patient is taking a class IA antiarrhythmic, check for these ECG changes:

- *QRS complex*—slightly widened; increased widening is an early sign of toxicity
- *T wave*—may be flattened or inverted
- *U wave*—may be present
- *QT interval*—prolonged.

Alert Because class IA antiarrhythmics prolong the QT interval, the patient is prone to polymorphic ventricular tachycardia (torsades de pointes). (See ECG effects of class IA antiarrhythmics, page 188.)

ECG EFFECTS OF CLASS IA ANTIARRHYTHMICS

Class IA antiarrhythmics—such as procainamide and quinidine—affect the cardiac cycle in specific ways and lead to specific electrocardiogram (ECG) changes, as shown here. These drugs:
◆ block sodium influx during phase 0, which depresses the rate of depolarization
◆ prolong repolarization and the duration of the action potential
◆ lengthen the refractory period
◆ decrease contractility.

ECG characteristics of class IA antiarrhythmics:

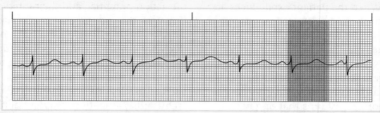

◆ QRS complex: slightly widened   ◆ QT interval: prolonged (shaded area)

CLASS IB

Class IB antiarrhythmics include lidocaine, mexiletine, tocainide, and phenytoin (rarely used). These agents interact rapidly with sodium channels, slowing phase 0 of the action potential and shortening phase 3. Class IB antiarrhythmics are used in suppressing life-threatening ventricular ectopy, ventricular tachycardia, and ventricular fibrillation.

ECG characteristics

When a patient is taking a class IB antiarrhythmic, check for these ECG changes:
● *PR interval*—may be prolonged
● *QT interval*—shortened. (See *ECG effects of class IB antiarrhythmics.*)\

CLASS IC

Class IC antiarrhythmics, including flecainide, propafenone, and moricizine (shares properties of classes IA, IB, and IC), interact slowly with sodium channels. Phase 0 is markedly slowed and conduction is decreased.

   Alert   *Class IC antiarrhythmics are generally reserved for patients with refractory supraventricular and ventricular arrhythmias because these drugs may cause or worsen arrhythmias.*

ECG characteristics

When a patient is taking a class IC antiarrhythmic, look for these ECG changes:
● *PR interval*—prolonged
● *QRS complex*—widened
● *QT interval*—prolonged. (See *ECG effects of class IC antiarrhythmics.*)

ECG EFFECTS OF CLASS IB ANTIARRHYTHMICS

Class IB antiarrhythmics—such as lidocaine and tocainide—may affect the QRS complex, as shown here. They may also:
- block sodium influx during phase 0, which depresses the rate of depolarization
- shorten repolarization and the duration of the action potential
- suppress ventricular automaticity in ischemic tissue.

Electrocardiogram (ECG) characteristics of class IB antiarrhythmics:

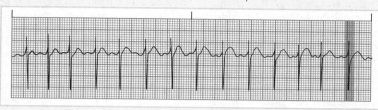

- *PR interval:* may be prolonged
- *QRS complex:* slightly widened (shaded area)

ECG EFFECTS OF CLASS IC ANTIARRHYTHMICS

Class IC antiarrhythmics—such as flecainide, moricizine, and propafenone—exert particular actions on the cardiac cycle and lead to specific electrocardiogram (ECG) changes, as shown here. These agents block sodium influx during phase 0, which depresses the rate of depolarization. Class IC antiarrhythmics exert no effect on repolarization or the duration of the action potential.

ECG characteristics of class IC antiarrhythmics:

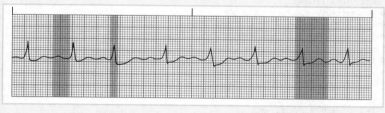

- *PR interval:* prolonged (shaded area, above left)
- *QRS complex:* widened (shaded area, above center)
- *QT interval:* prolonged (shaded area, above right)

Class II antiarrhythmics

Class II antiarrhythmics include drugs that reduce adrenergic activity in the heart. Beta-adrenergic antagonists, also called *beta-adrenergic blockers,* are class II antiarrhythmics and include such drugs as acebutolol, atenolol, esmolol, labetalol, metoprolol, and propranolol. Beta-adrenergic antagonists block beta receptors in the sympathetic nervous system. As a result, phase 4 depolarization is diminished, which leads to depressed automaticity of the sinoatrial node and increased atrial and atrioventricular (AV) node refractory periods.

Class II antiarrhythmics are used to treat supraventricular and ventricular arrhythmias, especially those caused by excess circulating catecholamines.

Beta-adrenergic blockers are classified according to their effects. Cardioselective beta-adrenergic blockers (such as metoprolol and atenolol) block only beta$_1$ receptors, which decrease heart rate, contractility, and conductivity. Noncardioselective beta-adrenergic blockers (such as propanolol and labetalol) block beta$_1$ and beta$_2$ receptors and may cause vasoconstriction and bronchospasm because they block beta$_2$ receptors that relax smooth muscle in the bronchi and blood vessels.

Alert *Use class II antiarrhythmics cautiously in patients with pulmonary disease, such as chronic obstructive pulmonary disease, because of the risk of bronchospasm.*

ECG CHARACTERISTICS

When a patient is taking a class II antiarrhythmic, look for these ECG changes:

ECG EFFECTS OF CLASS II ANTIARRHYTHMICS

Class II antiarrhythmics—including beta-adrenergic blockers such as acebutolol, esmolol, and propranolol—exert particular actions on the cardiac cycle and lead to specific electrocardiogram (ECG) changes, as shown here. These drugs:
◆ depress sinoatrial node automaticity
◆ shorten the duration of the action potential
◆ increase the refractory period of atrial and atrioventricular junctional tissues, which slows conduction
◆ inhibit sympathetic activity.

ECG characteristics of class II antiarrhythmics:

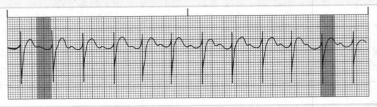

◆ *PR interval:* slightly prolonged (shaded area, above left)

◆ *QT interval:* slightly shortened (shaded area, above right)

- *Rate*—atrial and ventricular rates are decreased
- *PR interval*—slightly prolonged
- *QT interval*—slightly shortened. (See *ECG effects of class II antiarrhythmics*.)

Class III antiarrhythmics

Class III antiarrhythmics prolong the action potential duration, ultimately prolonging the effective refractory period. Class III drugs are called *potassium channel blockers* because they block the movement of potassium during phase 3 of the action potential. Drugs in this class include amiodarone, dofetilide, ibutilide, and sotalol (a nonselective beta-adrenergic blocker with mainly class III properties). All class III drugs have proarrhythmic po-

tential. Amiodarone is used to treat rapid atrial arrhythmias and ventricular arrhythmias. Dofetilide is used to treat atrial fibrillation. Ibutilide is used to rapidly convert recent-onset atrial fibrillation or atrial flutter to normal sinus rhythm. Sotalol is used to treat atrial and ventricular arrhythmias.

ECG CHARACTERISTICS

When a patient is taking a class III antiarrhythmic, look for these ECG changes:
- *PR interval*—prolonged
- *QRS complex*—widened
- *QT interval*—prolonged. (See *ECG effects of class III antiarrhythmics*.)

ECG EFFECTS OF CLASS III ANTIARRHYTHMICS

Class III antiarrhythmics—such as amiodarone, ibutilide, and sotalol—affect the cardiac cycle and cause electrocardiogram (ECG) changes, as shown here. These drugs:
- ◆ block potassium movement during phase 3
- ◆ increase the duration of the action potential
- ◆ prolong the effective refractory period.

ECG characteristics of class III antiarrhythmics:

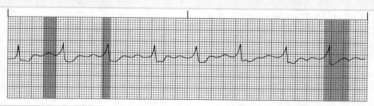

- ◆ PR interval: prolonged (shaded area, above left)
- ◆ QRS complex: widened (shaded area, above center)
- ◆ QT interval: prolonged (shaded area, above right)

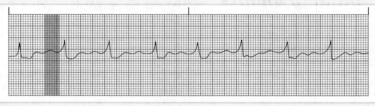
Class IV antiarrhythmics

Class IV antiarrhythmics block the
movement of calcium during phase 2
of the action potential. Because phase
2 is also called the *calcium channel* or
the *slow channel,* drugs that affect
phase 2 are also known as *calcium
channel blockers* or *slow channel blockers.*
Class IV antiarrhythmics slow conduction and increase the refractory period of calcium-dependent tissues, including the AV node. Drugs in this
class include diltiazem and verapamil
and are used to treat paroxysmal
supraventricular tachycardia, atrial
flutter and atrial fibrillation, and multifocal atrial tachycardia.

ECG CHARACTERISTICS

When a patient is taking a class IV
antiarrhythmic, look for these ECG
changes:
● *Rate*—atrial and ventricular rates—
decreased
● *PR interval*—prolonged. (See *ECG
effects of class IV antiarrhythmics.*)

Digoxin

Digoxin, the most commonly used
cardiac glycoside, works by inhibiting the enzyme adenosine triphos-
phatase. This enzyme is found in
the plasma membrane and acts as a
pump to exchange sodium ions for
potassium ions. Inhibition of sodium-
potassium–activated adenosine tri-
phosphatase enhances the movement
of calcium from the extracellular space
to the intracellular space, thereby

ECG EFFECTS OF DIGOXIN

Digoxin affects the cardiac cycle in various ways and may lead to the electrocardiogram (ECG) changes shown here.

ECG characteristics of digoxin:

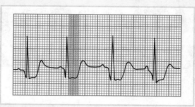

◆ ST segment: gradual sloping, causing ST-segment depression in the opposite direction of the QRS deflection (shaded area)

◆ P wave: may be notched

---

strengthening myocardial contractions.

The effects of digoxin on the electrical properties of the heart include direct and autonomic effects. *Direct effects* result in shortening of the action potential, which contributes to shortening of atrial and ventricular refractoriness. *Autonomic effects* involve the sympathetic and parasympathetic systems, enhancing vagal tone and slowing conduction through the SA and AV nodes. The drug also exerts an antiarrhythmic effect.

Digoxin is indicated in the treatment of heart failure, paroxysmal supraventricular tachycardia, and atrial flutter and atrial fibrillation.

ECG CHARACTERISTICS

When a patient is taking digoxin, look for these ECG changes:
- *Rate*—atrial and ventricular rates—decreased
- *PR interval*—prolonged
- *T wave*—decreased
- *ST segment*—shortened and depressed; sagging (scooping or sloping) of the segment is characteristic
- *P wave*—may be notched
- *QT interval*—shortened due to the shortened ST segment. (See *ECG effects of digoxin.*)

Alert *Digoxin has narrow window of therapeutic effectiveness and, at toxic levels, may cause numerous arrhythmias, including paroxysmal atrial tachycardia with block, AV block, atrial and junctional tachyarrhythmias, and ventricular arrhythmias.*

15

NONPHARMACOLOGIC TREATMENTS FOR ARRHYTHMIAS

Nonpharmacologic interventions for arrhythmias produce distinctive electrocardiogram (ECG) tracings. These interventions include various types of pacemakers, implantable cardioverter-defibrillators, radiofrequency ablation, and ventricular assist devices.

Pacemakers

A *pacemaker* is an artificial device that electrically stimulates the myocardium to depolarize, starting mechanical contractions. It works by generating an impulse from a power source and transmitting that impulse to the heart muscle. The impulse flows throughout the heart and causes the heart muscle to depolarize.

A pacemaker may be used when a patient has an arrhythmia, such as certain bradyarrhythmias and tachyarrhythmias, sick sinus syndrome (SSS), or second- and third-degree atrioventricular (AV) block. The device may be used as a temporary measure or a permanent one, depending on the patient's condition. Pacemakers are typically necessary after myocardial infarction or cardiac surgery.

This section examines how pacemakers work, ECG characteristics,

pacemaker programming, types of pacemakers, pacemaker function assessment, troubleshooting pacemaker problems, interventions, and patient teaching.

PACEMAKER COMPONENTS

A typical pacemaker has three main components: a pulse generator, pacing leads or wires, and one or more electrodes at the distal ends of leadwires. The *pulse generator* contains the pacemaker's power source and circuitry. It creates an electrical impulse that moves through the pacing leads to the electrodes, transmitting that impulse to the heart muscle and causing the heart to depolarize. The lithium battery in a permanent or implanted pacemaker serves as its power source and lasts between 5 and 10 years. A microchip in the device guides heart pacing.

A temporary pacemaker, which isn't implanted, is about the size of a small radio or telemetry box and is powered by alkaline batteries. These units also contain a microchip and are programmed by a touch pad or dials.

An electrical stimulus from the pulse generator moves through wires, or *pacing leads,* to the electrode tips. The leads for a pacemaker, designed

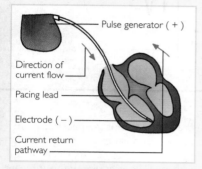
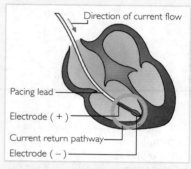
to stimulate a single heart chamber, are placed in either the atrium or the ventricle. For dual-chamber (or AV) pacing, the leads are placed in both chambers, usually on the right side of the heart. (See *Understanding pacing leads*.)

The *electrodes*—one on a unipolar lead or two on a bipolar lead—send information about electrical impulses in the myocardium back to the pulse generator. The pulse generator senses the heart's electrical activity and responds according to how it was programmed. A *unipolar lead system* is more sensitive to the heart's intrinsic electrical activity, such as skeletal muscle contraction or magnetic fields, than is a *bipolar system*. In addition, a bipolar system is more difficult to implant.

ECG CHARACTERISTICS

The most prominent characteristic of a pacemaker on an ECG is the *pacemaker spike*. (See *Identifying pacemaker spikes*, page 196.) It occurs when the pacemaker sends an electrical impulse to the heart muscle. The impulse appears as a vertical line, or spike. The collective group of spikes on an ECG is called *pacemaker artifact*.

Depending on the electrode's position, the spike appears in different locations on the waveform.

● When the pacemaker stimulates the atria, the spike is followed by a P wave and the patient's baseline QRS complex and T wave. This series of waveforms represents successful pacing, or *capture*, of the myocardium. The P wave appears different from the patient's normal P wave.

● When the pacemaker stimulates the ventricles, the spike is followed by

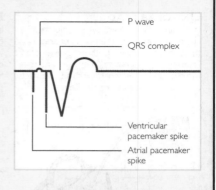
a QRS complex and a T wave. The QRS complex appears wider than the patient's own QRS complex because of how the pacemaker depolarizes the ventricles.

● When the pacemaker stimulates both the atria and ventricles, the spike is followed by a P wave, then a spike, and then a QRS complex. Be aware that the type of pacemaker and the patient's condition may affect whether every beat is paced.

PACEMAKER PROGRAMMING

Pacemakers are commonly known by their programmed function and by the number of heart chambers that have a pacing lead. Common programmable functions include rate, mode, output, sensitivity, AV interval, and upper and lower rate limits.

Synchronous and asynchronous pacing

Pacemakers can be classified according to sensitivity. In synchronous (*demand*) pacing, the pacemaker starts electrical impulses only when the heart's intrinsic heart rate falls below

the preset rate of the pacemaker. In asynchronous (*fixed*) pacing, the pacemaker constantly starts electrical impulses at a preset rate without regard to the patient's intrinsic electrical activity or heart rate. This type of pacemaker is rarely used.

Pacemaker description codes

The capabilities of permanent pacemakers are described by a five-letter coding system, although three or four letters are more commonly used. (See *Pacemaker coding system.*)

Pacing modes

A pacemaker's mode indicates its functions. Several different modes may be used during pacing, and they may not mimic the normal cardiac cycle. A three-letter code, rather than a five-letter code, is typically used to describe pacemaker function. Modes include AAI, VVI, DVI, and DDD. (See *AAI and VVI pacemakers,* page 198.)

AAI mode

The AAI (*atrial demand*) pacemaker is a single-chambered device that paces and senses the atria. When the pacemaker senses intrinsic atrial activity, it inhibits pacing and resets itself.

Because AAI pacemakers require a functioning AV node and an intact conduction system, they aren't used in AV block. An AAI pacemaker may be used in patients with sinus bradycardia, which may occur after cardiac surgery, or with SSS, as long as the AV node and His-Purkinje system aren't diseased.

VVI mode

The VVI (*ventricular demand*) pacemaker paces and senses the ventricles. When it senses intrinsic ventricular activity, it inhibits pacing. This single-chambered pacemaker benefits patients with complete heart block and those needing intermittent pacing. Because it doesn't affect atrial activity, it's used for patients who don't need an atrial kick—the extra 15% to 30% of cardiac output that comes from atrial contraction.

If a patient has spontaneous atrial activity, a VVI pacemaker won't synchronize the ventricular activity with it, so tricuspid and mitral insufficiency may develop. Patients who are sedentary may receive this pacemaker, but it

AAI AND VVI PACEMAKERS

AAI and VVI pacemakers are single-chamber pacemakers. The electrode is placed in the atrium for an AAI pacemaker; in the ventricle for a VVI pacemaker. The rhythm strips here show how each pacemaker works.

AAI PACEMAKER

An AAI pacemaker senses and paces only the atria. As shown in the shaded area below, a P wave follows each atrial spike (atrial depolarization). The QRS complexes reflect the heart's own conduction.

This pacemaker requires a functioning atrioventricular node and intact conduction system. It may be used in patients who have symptom-producing sinus bradycardia or sick sinus syndrome.

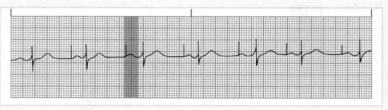

VVI PACEMAKER

A VVI pacemaker senses and paces the ventricles. When each spike is followed by a QRS complex (depolarization), as shown below, the rhythm is said to reflect 100% capture.

This pacemaker may be used in patients who have chronic atrial fibrillation with slow ventricular response and those who need infrequent pacing.

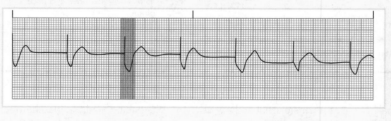

won't adjust its rate for patients who are more active.

DVI mode

The DVI, or *AV sequential,* pacemaker paces the atria and ventricles. (See *DVI pacemakers.*) However, this dual-chambered pacemaker senses only the ventricles' intrinsic activity, inhibiting ventricular pacing.

Two types of DVI pacemakers may be used—a committed DVI or a non-committed DVI. The *committed DVI pacemaker* doesn't sense intrinsic activity during the AV interval (the time between an atrial and ventricular spike). It generates an impulse even with spontaneous ventricular depolarization. The *noncommitted DVI pacemaker* is inhibited if a spontaneous depolarization occurs.

The DVI pacemaker helps patients with AV block or SSS who have a dis-

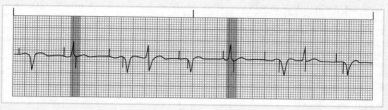
eased His-Purkinje conduction system. It provides the benefits of AV synchrony and atrial kick, thus improving cardiac output. However, it can't vary the atrial rate and isn't helpful in atrial fibrillation because it can't capture the atria. In addition, it may needlessly fire or inhibit its own pacing.

DDD mode

A DDD (*universal*) pacemaker is used with severe AV block. (See *DDD pacemakers,* page 200.) However, because the pacemaker possesses so many capabilities, it may be hard to troubleshoot problems.

Advantages of the DDD pacemaker include its:
- versatility
- programmability
- ability to change modes automatically

- ability to mimic the normal physiologic cardiac cycle, maintaining AV synchrony
- ability to sense and pace the atria and ventricles at the same time according to the intrinsic atrial rate and maximal rate limit.

Unlike other pacemakers, the DDD pacemaker is set with a rate range, rather than a single critical rate. It senses atrial activity and ensures that the ventricles respond to each atrial stimulation, thereby maintaining normal AV synchrony.

The DDD pacemaker fires when the ventricle doesn't respond on its own, and it paces the atria when the atrial rate falls below the lower set rate. In a patient with a high atrial rate, a safety mechanism allows the pacemaker to follow the intrinsic atrial rate only to a preset upper limit. That limit is usually set at about 130 beats/

DDD PACEMAKERS

When evaluating the rhythm strip of a patient with a DDD (universal) pacemaker, keep several points in mind.
◆ If the patient has an adequate intrinsic rhythm, the pacemaker won't fire; it doesn't need to.
◆ If you see an intrinsic P wave followed by a ventricular pacemaker spike, the pacemaker is tracking the atrial rate and assuring a ventricular response.
◆ If you see a pacemaker spike before a P wave, followed by an intrinsic ventricular QRS complex, the atrial rate is falling below the lower rate limit, causing the atrial channel to fire. Normal conduction to the ventricles follows.
◆ If you see a pacemaker spike before a P wave and before the QRS complex, no intrinsic activity is taking place in either the atria or ventricles.

In the rhythm strip shown below, complexes 1, 2, 4, and 7 show the atrial-synchronous mode, set at a rate of 70. The patient has an intrinsic P wave, so the pacemaker only ensures that the ventricles respond. Complexes 3, 5, 8, 10, and 12 are intrinsic ventricular depolarizations. The pacemaker senses them and doesn't fire. In complexes 6, 9, and 11, the pacemaker is pacing the atria and ventricles in sequence. In complex 13, only the atria are paced; the ventricles respond on their own.

Electrocardiogram characteristic of DDD pacemakers:

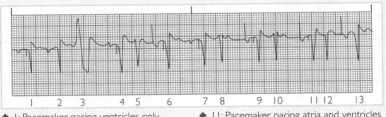

◆ 1: Pacemaker pacing ventricles only   ◆ 11: Pacemaker pacing atria and ventricles

minute and helps to prevent the ventricles from responding to atrial tachycardia or atrial flutter.

TYPES OF PACEMAKERS

A pacemaker can be permanent or temporary. Certain pacemakers can pace both the left and right ventricles.

Permanent pacemakers

A *permanent pacemaker* is used to treat chronic heart conditions, such as second- and third-degree AV block. It's surgically implanted, usually under local anesthesia. The leads are placed transvenously, positioned in the appropriate chambers, and then anchored to the endocardium. (See *Placing a permanent pacemaker*.)

The generator is then implanted in a subcutaneous pocket of tissue usually constructed under the patient's clavicle. Most permanent pacemakers are programmed before implantation. The programming sets the conditions under which the pacemaker functions, and can be adjusted externally, if necessary.

Biventricular pacemakers

Biventricular pacing, also referred to as *cardiac resynchronization therapy,* is used to treat patients with moderate and severe heart failure who have left ventricular dyssynchrony. These patients

PLACING A PERMANENT PACEMAKER

Implanting a pacemaker is a surgical procedure performed with local anesthesia and moderate sedation. To implant an endocardial pacemaker, the surgeon usually selects a transvenous route and begins lead placement by inserting a catheter percutaneously or by venous cutdown. Then using fluoroscopic guidance, the surgeon threads the catheter through the vein until the tip reaches the endocardium.

LEAD PLACEMENT

For lead placement in the atrium, the tip must lodge in the right atrium or coronary sinus, as shown here. For placement in the ventricle, it must lodge in the right ventricular apex in one of the interior muscular ridges, or trabeculae.

IMPLANTING THE GENERATOR

When the lead is in proper position, the surgeon secures the pulse generator in a subcutaneous pocket of tissue just below the patient's clavicle. Changing the generator's battery or microchip circuitry requires only a shallow incision over the site and a quick exchange of components.

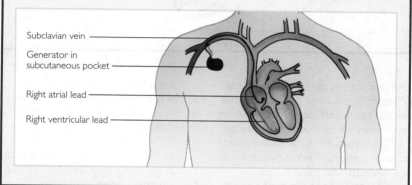

Subclavian vein

Generator in subcutaneous pocket

Right atrial lead

Right ventricular lead

have intraventricular conduction defects, which cause uncoordinated contraction of the right and left ventricles and a wide QRS complex on an ECG. Left ventricular dyssynchrony has been associated with worsening heart failure and increased morbidity and mortality.

Under normal conditions, the right and left ventricles contract simultaneously to pump blood to the lungs and body, respectively. However, in a patient with heart failure, the damaged ventricles can't pump as forcefully, and the amount of blood ejected with each contraction is reduced. If the ventricular conduction pathways are also damaged, electrical impulses reach the ventricles at different times, producing asynchronous contractions (intraventricular conduction defect), which further reduces the amount of blood that the heart pumps, worsening the patient's symptoms.

To compensate for this reduced cardiac output, the sympathetic nervous system releases *neurohormones,* such as aldosterone, norepinephrine, and vasopressin, to boost the amount of blood ejected with each contraction. The resultant tachycardia and vasoconstriction increase the heart's

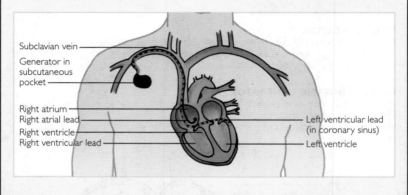

BIVENTRICULAR LEAD PLACEMENT

The biventricular pacemaker uses three leads: one to pace the right atrium, one to pace the right ventricle, and one to pace the left ventricle. The left ventricular lead is placed in the coronary sinus. Both ventricles are paced at the same time, causing them to contract simultaneously, thereby improving cardiac output.

Subclavian vein

Generator in subcutaneous pocket

Right atrium
Right atrial lead
Right ventricle
Right ventricular lead

Left ventricular lead (in coronary sinus)
Left ventricle

demand for oxygen, reduce diastolic filling time, promote sodium and water retention, and increase the pressure against which the heart must pump.

To coordinate ventricular contractions and improve hemodynamic status, biventricular pacemakers use three leads—one in the right atrium, and one in each ventricle. Both ventricles are paced at the same time, causing them to contract simultaneously, thereby increasing cardiac output.

Unlike traditional lead placement, the electrode tip for the left ventricle is placed in the coronary sinus to a branch of the inferior cardiac vein. Because this electrode tip isn't anchored in place, lead displacement may occur. (See *Biventricular lead placement*.)

Biventricular pacing produces an immediate improvement in the patient's symptoms and activity tolerance. Moreover, biventricular pacing improves left ventricular remodeling and diastolic function and reduces sympathetic stimulation. This slows the progression of heart failure and improves quality of life for many patients.

Keep in mind, however, that not all patients with heart failure benefit from biventricular pacing. Candidates should have both systolic heart failure and ventricular dyssynchrony along with these characteristics:
● symptom-producing heart failure despite maximal medical therapy
● moderate to severe heart failure (New York Heart Association class III or IV)
● QRS complex greater than 0.13 second
● left ventricular ejection fraction of 35% or less.

Temporary pacemakers
A *temporary pacemaker* is typically inserted in an emergency. The patient

may show signs of decreased cardiac output, such as hypotension or syncope. The temporary pacemaker supports the patient until the condition resolves.

A temporary pacemaker also can serve as a bridge until a permanent pacemaker is inserted. These pacemakers are used for patients with high-grade heart block, bradycardia, or low cardiac output. Several types of temporary pacemakers are available, including transvenous, epicardial, transcutaneous, and transthoracic.

Transvenous pacemakers

Physicians usually use the transvenous approach (inserting the pacemaker through a vein, such as the subclavian or internal jugular vein) when placing a temporary pacemaker. The *transvenous pacemaker* is probably the most common and reliable type of temporary pacemaker. It's usually inserted at the bedside or in a fluoroscopy suite. The leadwires are advanced through a catheter into the right ventricle or atrium and then connected to the pulse generator.

Epicardial pacemakers

Epicardial pacemakers are commonly used for patients undergoing cardiac surgery. The tips of the leadwires are attached to the heart's surface and the wires are brought through the chest wall, below the incision where they're attached to the pulse generator. The leadwires are usually removed several days after surgery, or when the patient no longer requires them.

Transcutaneous pacemakers

A transcutaneous (*external*) pacemaker is commonly used in emergencies until a transvenous pacemaker can be inserted. In this noninvasive method, there are two placement positions for the electrode pads.

- Anterior-posterior placement (most common):
– Place the anterior (front) electrode pad on the patient's anterior chest wall to the left of the sternum at the fourth and fifth intercostal spaces, halfway between the xiphoid process and left nipple.
– Place the posterior (back) electrode pad on the left side of the back directly behind the anterior pad, just below the scapula to the left of the spine.
- Anterior-apex placement (alternative placement, if the patient can't tolerate posterior placement):
– Place the anterior (front) electrode pad on the patient's anterior chest wall to the left of the sternum at the fourth and fifth intercostal spaces, midaxillary line.
– Place the posterior (back) electrode pad on the patient's anterior chest wall to the right of the upper sternum below the clavicle at the second or third intercostal space.

An external pulse generator then emits pacing impulses that travel through the patient's skin to the heart muscle. Transcutaneous pacing is built into many defibrillators for use in emergencies. Transcutaneous pacemakers also have electrodes built into the same pads used for defibrillation.

Transcutaneous pacing is a quick, effective method of pacing heart rhythm. However, some patients may not be able to tolerate the irritating sensations produced from prolonged pacing at the levels needed to pace the heart externally. If the patient is hemodynamically stable, he may require sedation.

Transthoracic pacemakers

A *transthoracic pacemaker* is a type of ventricular pacemaker only used as a

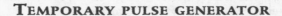

TEMPORARY PULSE GENERATOR

The settings on a temporary pulse generator may be changed in various ways to meet the patient's specific needs. The illustration below shows a single-chamber temporary pulse generator and gives brief descriptions of its various parts.

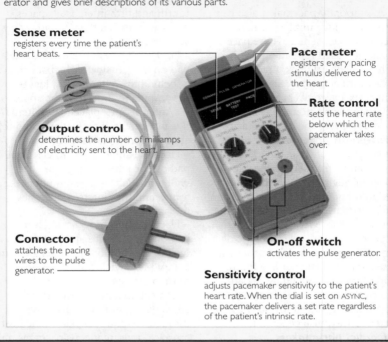

Sense meter
registers every time the patient's heart beats.

Pace meter
registers every pacing stimulus delivered to the heart.

Rate control
sets the heart rate below which the pacemaker takes over.

Output control
determines the number of milliamps of electricity sent to the heart.

Connector
attaches the pacing wires to the pulse generator.

On-off switch
activates the pulse generator.

Sensitivity control
adjusts pacemaker sensitivity to the patient's heart rate. When the dial is set on ASYNC, the pacemaker delivers a set rate regardless of the patient's intrinsic rate.

last resort during cardiac emergencies. Transthoracic pacing requires insertion of a long needle into the right ventricle, using a subxiphoid approach. A pacing wire is then guided directly into the endocardium.

Temporary pacemaker settings

A temporary pacemaker has several types of settings on the pulse generator. The rate control regulates how many impulses are generated in 1 minute and is measured in pulses per minute (ppm). The rate is usually set at 60 to 80 ppm. (See *Temporary pulse generator.*) The pacemaker fires if the patient's heart rate falls below the preset rate. The rate may be set higher if the patient has a tachyarrhythmia that's being treated with overdrive pacing.

A pacemaker's energy output is measured in milliamperes, a measurement that represents the stimulation threshold, or how much energy is required to stimulate the cardiac muscle to depolarize. The stimulation threshold is sometimes referred to as *energy required for capture.* The milliamperage is usually set between 10 mA and 20 mA.

You also can program the pacemaker's sensitivity, measured in millivolts. Most pacemakers allow the patient's heart to function naturally and assist only when necessary. The sensing threshold allows the pacemaker to do this by sensing the heart's normal activity.

EVALUATING PACEMAKER FUNCTION

After a pacemaker has been implanted, its function should be assessed. First, determine the pacemaker's mode and settings. If the patient had a permanent pacemaker implanted before admission, ask whether the wallet card from the manufacturer notes the mode and settings.

If the pacemaker was recently implanted, check the patient's medical record for information about the pacemaker settings—this precaution will help prevent misinterpretation of the ECG tracing. For instance, if the tracing has ventricular spikes but no atrial pacing spikes, you might assume that it's a VVI pacemaker when it could be a DVI pacemaker that has lost its atrial output.

Next, review the patient's 12-lead ECG. If it isn't available, examine lead V_1 or MCL_1 instead.

Select a monitoring lead that clearly shows the pacemaker spikes. Make sure the lead you select doesn't cause the cardiac monitor to misinterpret a spike for a QRS complex and double-count the heart rate. This misinterpretation may cause the alarm to sound, falsely signaling a high heart rate.

When looking at an ECG tracing for a patient with a pacemaker, consider the pacemaker mode, and then interpret the paced rhythm. Does it correlate with what you know about the pacemaker?

Look for information that tells you which chamber is paced. Is there capture? Is there a P wave or QRS complex after each atrial or ventricular spike? Or do the P waves and QRS complexes stem from intrinsic electrical activity?

Look for information about the pacemaker's sensing ability. If intrinsic atrial or ventricular activity is present, what's the pacemaker's response?

Look at the rate. What's the pacing rate per minute? Is it appropriate, given the pacemaker settings? Although you can determine the rate quickly by counting the number of complexes in a 6-second ECG strip, a more accurate method is to count the number of small boxes between complexes and divide this number into 1,500.

Knowing your patient's medical history and whether a pacemaker has been implanted will also help you to determine whether your patient is experiencing ventricular ectopy or paced activity on the ECG. (See *Distinguishing intermittent ventricular pacing from PVCs*, page 206.)

TROUBLESHOOTING PACEMAKER PROBLEMS

A malfunctioning pacemaker can lead to arrhythmias, hypotension, syncope, and other signs and symptoms of decreased cardiac output. (See *Recognizing a malfunctioning pacemaker*, pages 207 and 208.) Common problems with pacemakers that can lead to low cardiac output and loss of AV synchrony include:
- failure to capture
- failure to pace
- undersensing
- oversensing.

DISTINGUISHING INTERMITTENT VENTRICULAR PACING FROM PVCs

Knowing whether your patient has an artificial pacemaker will help you avoid mistaking a ventricular paced beat for a premature ventricular contraction (PVC). If your facility uses a monitoring system that eliminates artifact, make sure the monitor is set up correctly for a patient with a pacemaker. Otherwise, the pacemaker spikes may be eliminated as well.

If your patient has intermittent ventricular pacing, the paced ventricular complex will have a pacemaker spike preceding it, as shown in the shaded area of the top electrocardiogram (ECG) strip. You may need to look in different leads for a bipolar pacemaker spike because it's small and may be difficult to see. What's more, the paced ventricular complex of a properly functioning pacemaker won't occur early or prematurely; it will occur only when the patient's own ventricular rate falls below the rate set for the pacemaker.

If your patient is having PVCs, they won't have pacemaker spikes preceding them. Examples are shown in the shaded areas of the bottom ECG strip.

Intermittent ventricular pacing

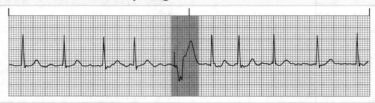

PVCs

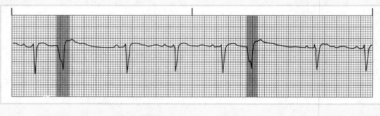

Failure to capture

Failure to capture appears on an ECG as a pacemaker spike without the appropriate atrial or ventricular response— a spike without a complex. Think of "failure to capture" as the pacemaker's inability to stimulate the chamber.

Causes of failure to capture include acidosis, electrolyte imbalances, fibrosis, incorrect leadwire position, a low mA or output setting, low battery, a broken or cracked leadwire, or perforation of the leadwire through the myocardium.

Failure to pace

Failure to pace is indicated by no pacemaker activity on an ECG when activity is expected. This problem may be caused by battery or circuit failure, cracked or broken leads, or interference between atrial and ventricular

Recognizing a Malfunctioning Pacemaker

Occasionally, pacemakers fail to function properly. When this happens, you'll need to take immediate action to correct the problem. The rhythm strips below show examples of problems that can occur with a temporary or permanent pacemaker.

FAILURE TO CAPTURE

◆ Electrocardiogram (ECG) shows a pacemaker spike without the appropriate atrial or ventricular response (spike without a complex), as shown at right.

◆ Patient may be asymptomatic or have signs of decreased cardiac output.

◆ Pacemaker can't stimulate the chamber.

◆ Problem may be caused by increased pacing thresholds related to certain situations:
– Metabolic or electrolyte imbalance
– Antiarrhythmics
– Fibrosis or edema at electrode tip

◆ Problem may be caused by lead malfunction:
– Dislodged lead
– Broken or damaged lead
– Perforation of myocardium by lead
– Loose connection between lead and pulse generator

◆ Related interventions may solve the problem:
– Treat metabolic disturbance.
– Replace damaged lead.
– Change pulse generator battery.
– Slowly increase output setting on the temporary pacemaker until capture occurs.
– Determine electrode placement with a chest X-ray, if needed.

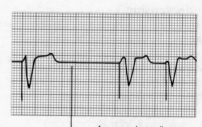

There's a pacemaker spike but no response from the heart.

FAILURE TO PACE

◆ ECG shows no pacemaker activity when pacemaker activity should be evident, as shown at right.

◆ Magnet application yields no response. (It should cause asynchronous pacing.)

◆ Problem has several common causes, including:
– depleted battery
– circuit failure
– lead malfunction
– inappropriate programming of sensing function
– electromagnetic interference.

◆ Failure to pace can lead to asystole or a severe decrease in cardiac output in the patient who is pacemaker dependent.

◆ If you think a pacemaker is failing to pace, you should place a temporary pacemaker (transcutaneous or transvenous) to prevent asystole.

◆ Related interventions may solve the problem:
– Replace pulse generator battery.
– Replace pulse generator unit.
– Adjust sensitivity setting.
– Remove source of electromagnetic interference.

A pacemaker spike should appear here but doesn't.

(continued)

FAILURE TO SENSE INTRINSIC BEATS (UNDERSENSING)

◆ ECG may show pacing spikes anywhere in the cycle, as shown at right.
◆ A pacemaker spike may appear where intrinsic cardiac activity is present.
◆ Patient may report feeling palpitations or skipped beats.
◆ Spikes are especially dangerous if they fall on the T wave because ventricular tachycardia or fibrillation may result.
◆ Problem has several common causes, including:
– battery failure
– fracture of pacing leadwire
– displacement of electrode tip
– "cross-talk" between atrial and ventricular channels
– electromagnetic interference mistaken for intrinsic signals.
◆ Related interventions may solve the problem:
– Replace the pulse generator battery.
– Replace the leadwires.
– Adjust the sensitivity setting.

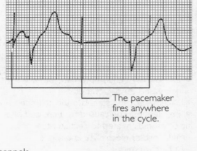

The pacemaker fires anywhere in the cycle.

sensing in a dual-chambered pacemaker. Failure to pace can lead to asystole.

Undersensing

Undersensing is indicated by a pacemaker spike when intrinsic cardiac activity is present. In asynchronous pacemakers that have codes, such as VOO or DOO, undersensing is a programming limitation.

When undersensing occurs in synchronous pacemakers, pacing spikes occur on the ECG where they shouldn't. Although they may appear in any part of the cardiac cycle, the spikes are especially dangerous if they fall on the T wave, where they can cause ventricular tachycardia or ventricular fibrillation.

In synchronous pacemakers, undersensing may be caused by elec-

trolyte imbalances, disconnection or dislodgment of a lead, improper lead placement, increased sensing threshold from edema or fibrosis at the electrode tip, drug interactions, or a depleted pacemaker battery.

Oversensing

Oversensing occurs if the pacemaker is too sensitive, misinterpreting muscle movements or other events in the cardiac cycle as intrinsic cardiac electrical activity. Pacing won't occur when it's needed, and the heart rate and AV synchrony won't be maintained.

INTERVENTIONS

Make sure you're familiar with different types of pacemakers and how they function, so you'll feel more confident in an emergency. When caring for a patient with a pacemaker, follow these guidelines:

Permanent pacemakers

- Use a systematic approach to assess pacemaker function for problems.
  – Identify the mode.
  – Find out the base rate and upper rate limit (maximum tracking or sensor rate).
  – Determine if features such as mode switching or rate response are activated.
  – Find out if the device is a biventricular pacemaker.
  – Determine if patient is pacemaker-dependent.
  – Identify the patient's signs and symptoms.
- Evaluate all sources of information:
  – patient identification card issued by the pacemaker manufacturer
  – patient history
  – patient or family knowledge of device function
  – physician notes, printouts from programmer if available
  – ECG observation.
- Review the patient's 12-lead ECG to evaluate pacemaker function. If unavailable, examine lead V_1 or MCL_1 instead.
- Select a monitoring lead that clearly shows the pacemaker spikes and compare at least two leads to verify what you observe.
- Remember that visibility of spikes depends on pacing polarity and the type of lead.
- Measure the rate and interpret the paced rhythm.
- Compare the morphology of paced and intrinsic complexes (traditional right ventricular pacing should produce a morphology similar to left bundle-branch block pattern).
- Differentiate between ventricular ectopy and paced activity.
- Look for information about which chamber is paced and the pacemaker's sensing function.
- Monitor the patient's vital signs.
- Look for evidence of problems:
  – decreased cardiac output (hypotension, chest pain, dyspnea, syncope)
  – infection
  – pneumothorax
  – abnormal electrical stimulation occurring in synchrony with the pacemaker
  – pectoral muscle twitching
  – hiccups (stimulation of diaphragm)
  – cardiac tamponade.
- Know that placing a magnet over the pulse generator makes the pacemaker temporarily revert to an asynchronous mode (safety mode) at a preset rate. (See *Assessing pacemaker function,* page 210.)

Biventricular pacemakers

Provide the same basic care to the patient with a biventricular pacemaker that you would give a patient with a standard permanent pacemaker. Specific care includes these guidelines:

- Because of the position of the left ventricular lead, watch for stimulation of the diaphragm and left chest wall. Notify the practitioner if this occurs because the left ventricular lead may need repositioning.
- Observe the ECG for pacemaker spikes. Although both ventricles are paced, only one pacemaker spike is seen.
- Measure the duration of the QRS complex. Typically, you'll observe a narrowing of the QRS complex. A widened QRS complex may indicate

When you apply a magnet to a patient's pacemaker, the device reverts to a predefined (asynchronous) response mode that allows you to assess various aspects of pacemaker function. Specifically, you can:
◆ determine which chambers are being paced
◆ assess capture
◆ provide emergency pacing if the device malfunctions
◆ ensure pacing despite electromagnetic interference
◆ assess battery life by checking the magnet rate—a predetermined rate that indicates the need for battery replacement.

Keep in mind, however, that you must know which implanted device the patient has before you consider using a magnet on it. The patient might have an implantable cardioverter-defibrillator (ICD), which is only rarely an appropriate target for magnet application.

What's more, because pacemaker and ICDs are similar in generator size and implant location, it's not as easy to differentiate between the two. In addition, a single device may perform multiple functions.

In general, you shouldn't apply a magnet to an ICD or a pacemaker-ICD combination. Applying a magnet to an ICD can cause an unexpected response because various responses can be programmed or determined by the manufacturer. When directed, applying a magnet to an ICD usually suspends therapies for ventricular tachycardia and fibrillation while leaving bradycardia pacing active, which may be helpful in patients who receive multiple, inappropriate shocks. Some models may beep when exposed to a magnetic field.

---

that the left ventricular lead is no longer positioned properly.

Temporary pacemakers
● Check stimulation and sensing thresholds daily because they increase over time.
● Assess the pacemaker regularly to check for possible problems:
– failure to capture
– failure to pace
– undersensing
– oversensing.
● Turn or reposition the patient carefully to avoid dislodging the leadwire.
● Follow recommended electrical safety precautions.
● Avoid microshocks to the patient by making sure that the bed and all electrical equipment are grounded properly, and that all pacing wires and connections to temporary wires are insulated with moisture-proof material (such as a disposable glove).

● Obtain a chest X-ray and assist the practitioner with repositioning the leadwire, if required.

Alert All invasive temporary pacing has the potential to deliver a shock directly to the heart along the pacing wire, resulting in ventricular tachycardia or fibrillation.
● Defibrillation and cardioversion (up to 360 joules) don't usually require that the pulse generator be disconnected.
● Look for evidence of problems:
– decreased cardiac output (hypotension, chest pain, dyspnea, syncope)
– infection
– pneumothorax
– abnormal electrical stimulation occurring in synchrony with the pacemaker
– pectoral muscle twitching
– hiccups (stimulation of diaphragm)

- signs of a perforated ventricle and the resultant cardiac tamponade. Signs and symptoms include persistent hiccups, tachycardia, distant heart sounds, pulsus paradoxus (indicated by a drop in the strength of a pulse during inspiration), hypotension with narrowed pulse pressure, cyanosis, distended jugular veins, decreased urine output, restlessness, and complaints of fullness in the chest. Notify the practitioner immediately if you note any of these signs and symptoms.

● If there's no output (pacing is required but the pacemaker fails to stimulate the heart), take these steps:
– Verify that the pacemaker is on.
– Check the output settings.
– Change the pulse generator battery.
– Change the pulse generator.
– Check for disconnection or dislodgment of the pacing wire.

PATIENT TEACHING

Following pacemaker insertion, be sure to cover these points with the patient and his family.

Permanent pacemakers

● Provide information to the patient about:
– pacemaker's function
– related anatomy and physiology
– patient's indication for pacemaker
– postoperative care and routines.
● Provide discharge instructions, which usually include these topics:
– incision care
– signs of pocket complications (hematoma, infection, bleeding)
– avoidance of heavy lifting or vigorous activity for 2 to 4 weeks

– limited arm movement on side of pacemaker
– medical follow-up
– transtelephonic monitoring follow-up, if indicated
– identification card to be carried
– procedure for taking pulse.

● Explain signs and symptoms to report to practitioner:
– light-headedness, syncope, fatigue, palpitations, muscle stimulation, hiccups
– slow (below the base rate) or unusually fast heart rate.

● Because modern pacemakers are well shielded from environmental interactions, explain that the patient can safely use:
– most common household appliances, including microwaves
– cellular phones (on the opposite side of pacemaker)
– spark-ignited combustion engines (leaf blower, lawnmower, automobile)
– office equipment (computer, copier, fax machine)
– light shop equipment.

● Caution the patient to avoid close or prolonged exposure to potential sources of electromagnetic interference. (See *Understanding EMI*, page 212.)

● Remind the patient about travel-related issues:
– Metal detectors don't disturb pacemaker function, but may detect the device.
– Handheld scanning tools shouldn't be used over the pacemaker or near it.
– An identification card may be needed to show security personnel.

Biventricular pacemakers

Provide the same basic teaching that you would give to the patient receiving a permanent pacemaker. In addition, when a patient has a biventricular pacemaker, be sure to cover these points:
● Explain to the patient and his family why a biventricular pacemaker is needed, how it works, and what they can expect.
● Tell the patient and his family that it's sometimes difficult to place the left ventricular lead and that the procedure can take 3 hours or more.
● Stress the importance of calling the practitioner immediately if the patient develops chest pain, shortness of breath, swelling of the hands or feet, or a weight gain of 3 lb (1.4 kg) in 24 hours or 5 lb (2.3 kg) in 48 to 72 hours.

Temporary pacemakers

● Provide information to the patient about the temporary pacemaker's function, related anatomy and physiology, the need for the pacemaker,

and potential need for a permanent pacemaker.
● Explain postprocedure care and pain management.
● Advise the patient not to get out of bed without assistance.
● Instruct the patient not to manipulate the pacemaker wires or pulse generator.
● Explain symptoms to report, such as light-headedness, syncope, palpitations, muscle stimulation, or hiccups.
● Advise the patient to limit arm movement on the same side of the pacemaker.

Implantable cardioverter-defibrillator

An *implantable cardioverter-defibrillator* (ICD) is an electronic device implanted in the patient's body to provide continuous monitoring of the heart for bradycardia, ventricular tachycardia,

Understanding an ICD

An implantable cardioverter-defibrillator (ICD) consists of a pulse-generator box and a lead-wire system that incorporates either one or two leads. The system shown here includes a ventricular leadwire and an atrial leadwire. Features of the generator and lead wires are detailed below.

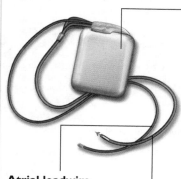

Pulse generator

◆ Is a small, battery-powered, programmable computer

◆ Monitors heart rate and rhythm

◆ Initiates the delivery of paced beats or defibrillatory shocks

◆ Stores information about the heart's activity before, during, and after an arrhythmia

◆ Tracks delivery and outcome of treatment

◆ Stores electrograms (similar to ECG strip when printed)

◆ Permits easy retrieval of all stored information

Atrial leadwire

◆ Is insulated

◆ Carries signals from the atrium to the pulse generator

◆ Delivers pacing impulses to the atrium

Ventricular leadwire

◆ Is insulated

◆ Carries signals from the ventricle to the pulse generator

◆ Delivers electrical energy from the pulse generator to the ventricle

---

and ventricular fibrillation. The device then administers either shocks or paced beats to treat the dangerous arrhythmia. In general, ICDs are indicated for patients for whom drug therapy, surgery, or catheter ablation has failed to prevent the arrhythmia.

An ICD consists of a programmable pulse generator and one or more leadwires. The pulse generator is a small battery-powered computer that monitors the heart's electrical signals and delivers electrical therapy when it identifies an abnormal rhythm. The leads are insulated wires that carry the heart signal to the pulse generator and deliver the electrical energy from the

pulse generator to the heart. (See *Understanding an ICD*.)

An ICD also stores information about the heart's activity before, during, and after an arrhythmia, along with tracking which treatment was delivered and the treatment's outcome. Many devices also store electrograms (electrical tracings similar to ECGs). With an interrogation device, a practitioner can retrieve this information to evaluate ICD function and battery status and to adjust ICD system settings.

Modern advanced devices can detect a wide range of arrhythmias and automatically respond with the appro-

Types of ICD therapies

An implantable cardioverter-defibrillator (ICD) can deliver a range of therapies depending on the type of device, how the device is programmed, and the arrhythmia it detects. Therapies include antitachycardia pacing, bradycardia pacing, cardioversion, and defibrillation.

THERAPY	DESCRIPTION
Antitachycardia pacing	A series of small, rapid, electrical pacing pulses are used to interrupt atrial fibrillation or ventricular tachycardia (VT) and return the heart to its normal rhythm. Antitachycardia pacing isn't appropriate for all patients and begins only after appropriate electrophysiology studies.
Bradycardia pacing	Electrical pacing pulses are used when natural electrical signals are too slow. ICDs can sense and pace one chamber (VVI pacing) of the heart at a preset rate, both chambers (DDD pacing), or function as a biventricular pacemaker.
Cardioversion	A low- or high-energy shock (up to 35 joules) is timed to the R wave to terminate VT and return the heart to its normal rhythm.
Defibrillation	A high-energy shock (up to 35 joules) is given to the heart to terminate ventricular fibrillation and return the heart to its normal rhythm.

priate therapy, such as bradycardia pacing (both single- and dual-chamber), antitachycardia pacing, cardioversion, and defibrillation. ICDs that provide therapy for atrial arrhythmias, such as atrial fibrillation, also are available. (See *Types of ICD therapies*.)

The procedure for ICD insertion is similar to that of a permanent pacemaker and may be done in a cardiac catheterization laboratory. Sometimes a patient who requires other surgery, such as coronary artery bypass grafting, may have the device implanted in the operating room. (See *Implantable cardioverter-defibrillator placement*.)

INTERVENTIONS

When caring for a patient with an ICD, it's important to know how the device is programmed. This information is available through a status report that can be obtained and printed by a practitioner or specially trained technician. This retrieval involves placing a specialized piece of equipment over the implanted pulse generator to retrieve pacing function. If the patient experiences an arrhythmia or the ICD delivers a therapy, the recorded program information helps to evaluate the functioning of the device (See *Analyzing ICD function*, page 216.)

Program information includes:
- type and model of ICD
- status of the device (on or off)
- detection rates
- therapies that will be delivered: pacing, antitachycardia pacing, cardioversion, and defibrillation.

If your patient experiences an arrhythmia:
- Assess the patient for signs and symptoms related to decreased cardiac output.
- Record the patient's ECG rhythm.
- Evaluate the appropriateness of any delivered ICD therapy.
- If the patient experiences cardiac arrest, start cardiopulmonary resusci-

IMPLANTABLE CARDIOVERTER-DEFIBRILLATOR PLACEMENT

A specially trained cardiologist implants the pulse generator and lead wires in the cardiac catheterization laboratory with the patient under local anesthesia. Occasionally, a patient who requires other surgery, such as coronary artery bypass, may have the device implanted in the operating room.

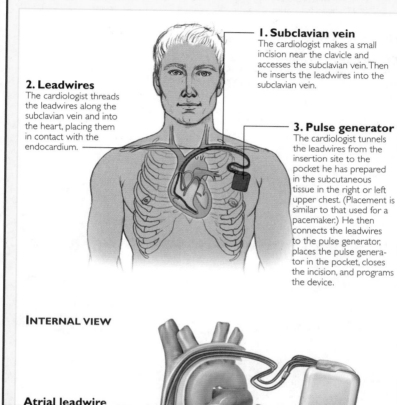

1. Subclavian vein
The cardiologist makes a small incision near the clavicle and accesses the subclavian vein. Then he inserts the leadwires into the subclavian vein.

2. Leadwires
The cardiologist threads the leadwires along the subclavian vein and into the heart, placing them in contact with the endocardium.

3. Pulse generator
The cardiologist tunnels the leadwires from the insertion site to the pocket he has prepared in the subcutaneous tissue in the right or left upper chest. (Placement is similar to that used for a pacemaker.) He then connects the leadwires to the pulse generator, places the pulse generator in the pocket, closes the incision, and programs the device.

INTERNAL VIEW

Atrial leadwire
Positioned so that the tip abuts the atrial endocardium

Ventricular leadwire
Has a fixation device that attaches to the ventricular endocardium

ANALYZING ICD FUNCTION

To evaluate the function of an implantable cardioverter-defibrillator (ICD), compare the monitor strips with the device status report. The example shown here demonstrates proper device functioning for ventricular tachycardia (VT) according to the programmed parameters. When VT occurs, the device is programmed to deliver antitachycardia pacing consisting of eight pacing stimuli six separate times. If the arrhythmia doesn't terminate or deteriorates to ventricular fibrillation, the device is programmed to deliver a cardioversion shock. This episode of VT converts to normal sinus rhythm with the first cardioversion.

STATUS REPORT

VT THERAPY	1	2	3	4
Therapy status	On	On	On	On
Therapy type	ATP	CV	CV	CV
Initial # pulses	8			
# Sequences	6			
Energy (J)		10	34	34
Waveform		Biphasic	Biphasic	Biphasic

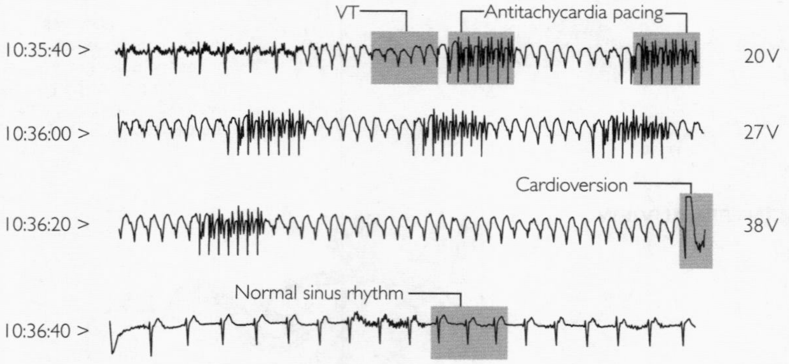

tation (CPR) and advanced cardiac life support.
● If the patient needs external defibrillation, position the paddles as far from the device as possible or use the anteroposterior paddle position.

PATIENT TEACHING
● Explain to the patient and his family why an ICD is needed, how it works, potential complications, and what they can expect. Make sure they also understand ICD terminology.
● Discuss signs and symptoms to report to the practitioner immediately.

- Advise the patient to wear a medical identification bracelet indicating ICD placement.
- Educate family members in emergency techniques (such as dialing 911 and performing CPR) in case the device fails.
- Explain that electrical or electronic devices may disrupt the device.
- Advise the patient to avoid placing excessive pressure over the insertion site, or moving or jerking the area until the postoperative visit.
- Tell the patient to follow normal routines, as allowed by the practitioner, and to increase exercise, as tolerated. After the first 24 hours, show the patient how to perform passive range-of-motion exercises, and progress, as tolerated.
- Remind the patient to carry information regarding his ICD at all times and to inform airline clerks as well as individuals performing diagnostic studies (such as computed tomography scans and magnetic resonance imaging).
- Stress the importance of follow-up care and checkups.

Radiofrequency ablation

Radiofrequency ablation is an invasive procedure that may be used to treat arrhythmias in patients who haven't responded to antiarrhythmics or cardioversion or who can't tolerate antiarrhythmics. In this procedure, a burst of radiofrequency energy is delivered through a catheter to the heart tissue to destroy the arrhythmia's focus or block the conduction pathway. Radiofrequency ablation is effective in treating patients with atrial fibrillation and flutter, ventricular tachycardia, AV nodal reentry tachycardia, and Wolff-Parkinson-White (WPW) syndrome.

The patient first undergoes electrophysiology studies to identify and map the specific area of the heart that's causing the arrhythmia. The ablation catheters are inserted into a vein (usually the femoral vein), and moved to the heart, where short bursts of radiofrequency waves destroy a small, targeted area of heart tissue. The destroyed tissue can no longer conduct electrical impulses. Other types of energy also may be used, such as microwave, sonar, or cryo (freezing). In some patients, the tissue inside the pulmonary vein is responsible for the arrhythmia. Targeted radiofrequency ablation is used to block these abnormal impulses. (See *Using radiofrequency ablation,* page 218.)

If a rapid arrhythmia that originates above the AV node (such as atrial fibrillation) isn't terminated by targeted ablation, AV nodal ablation may be used to block electrical impulses from being conducted to the ventricles. After ablation of the AV node, the patient may need a pacemaker because impulses can no longer be conducted from the atria to the ventricles. If the atria continue to beat irregularly, anticoagulation therapy also will be needed to reduce the risk of stroke.

If the patient has WPW syndrome, electrophysiology studies can locate the accessory pathway and ablation can destroy it. When reentry is the cause of the arrhythmia, such as AV nodal reentry tachycardia, ablation can destroy the pathway without affecting the AV node.

Using radiofrequency ablation

In radiofrequency ablation, special catheters are inserted in a vein and advanced to the heart. After the arrhythmia's source is identified, radiofrequency energy is used to destroy the source of the abnormal electrical impulses or abnormal conduction pathway.

AV NODAL ABLATION

If a rapid arrhythmia originates above the atrioventricular (AV) node, the radiofrequency ablation catheter is directed to the AV node where its energy is used to destroy the AV node to block impulses from reaching the ventricles.

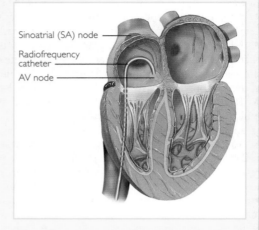

Sinoatrial (SA) node

Radiofrequency catheter

AV node

PULMONARY VEIN ABLATION

If the pulmonary vein is the source of the arrhythmia, the radiofrequency catheter is directed to the base of the pulmonary vein where its energy is used to destroy the tissue at the base of the pulmonary vein.

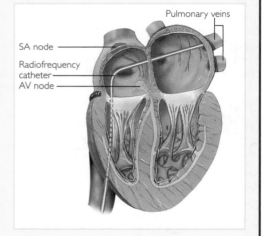

Pulmonary veins

SA node

Radiofrequency catheter

AV node

INTERVENTIONS

When caring for a patient after radiofrequency ablation, follow these guidelines:

● Provide continuous cardiac monitoring, assessing for arrhythmias and ischemic changes.

● Place the patient on bed rest for 8 hours, or as ordered, and keep the affected extremity straight. Maintain the head of the bed between 15 and 30 degrees.

● Assess the patient's vital signs every 15 minutes for the first hour, then every 30 minutes for 4 hours, unless the patient's condition warrants more frequent checking.

● Assess peripheral pulses distal to the catheter insertion site as well as the color, sensation, temperature, and capillary refill of the affected extremity.

● Check the catheter insertion site for bleeding or hematoma.

● Monitor the patient for complications, such as hemorrhage, stroke, perforation of the heart, arrhythmias, phrenic nerve damage, pericarditis, pulmonary vein stenosis or thrombosis, or sudden death.

PATIENT TEACHING

● Discuss with the patient and his family why radiofrequency ablation is needed, how it works, and what they can expect.

● If electrophysiology studies are to be done first, explain to the patient and his family that the procedure can take up to 6 hours.

● Explain that the patient may be hospitalized for 24 to 48 hours to monitor his heart rhythm.

● Provide pacemaker teaching if the patient had a pacemaker inserted.

Ventricular assist devices

Ventricular assist devices (VADs) are designed to decrease the heart's workload and increase cardiac output in patients with ventricular failure. Left ventricular, right ventricular, and biventricular VADs are available. (See *How VAD helps a failing heart,* page 220.)

Because a VAD supports the heart's pumping function rather than altering electrical function, it doesn't affect the heart's electrical activity. As a result, you probably won't see ECG changes caused by the VAD.

VADs may be indicated for patients who can't be weaned from cardiopulmonary bypass or intra-aortic balloon pump as well as for patients who are awaiting heart transplantation.

In a surgical procedure, blood is diverted from a ventricle to an artificial pump, which maintains systemic perfusion. VADs are commonly used as a bridge to maintain perfusion until a heart transplantation procedure can be performed.

A VAD is used to provide systemic or pulmonary support, or both:

● A right VAD provides pulmonary support by diverting blood from the failing right ventricle to the VAD, which then pumps the blood to the pulmonary circulation by way of the VAD connection to the pulmonary artery.

● With a left VAD, blood flows from the left ventricle to the VAD, which then pumps blood back to the body by way of the VAD connection to the aorta.

How VAD helps a failing heart

A ventricular assist device (VAD), which is commonly called a *bridge to transplant*, is a mechanical pump that relieves the ventricle's workload as the heart heals or until a donor heart is located.

IMPLANTABLE
The typical VAD is implanted in the upper abdominal wall. An inflow cannula drains blood from the left ventricle into a pump, which then pushes the blood into the aorta through the outflow cannula.

PUMP OPTIONS
VADs are available as continuous-flow or pulsatile pumps. A *continuous-flow pump* fills continuously and returns blood to the aorta at a constant rate. A *pulsatile pump* may work in one of two ways: It may fill during systole and pump blood into the aorta during diastole, or it may pump irrespective of the patient's cardiac cycle.

Many types of VAD systems are available. The illustration below shows a VAD implanted in the left abdominal wall.

POTENTIAL COMPLICATIONS
Despite the use of anticoagulants, the VAD may cause thrombi formation, leading to pulmonary embolism, transient ischemic attack, or stroke. Other complications may include heart failure, bleeding, cardiac tamponade, infection, sepsis, or device failure.

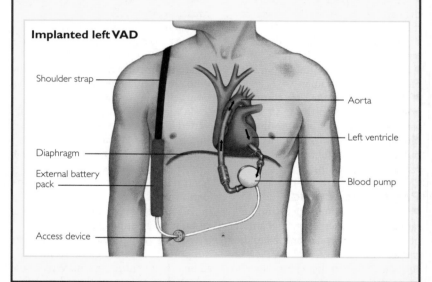

Implanted left VAD

Shoulder strap

Diaphragm

External battery pack

Access device

Aorta

Left ventricle

Blood pump

- When biventricular support is needed, both may be used.

INTERVENTIONS
When caring for a patient with a VAD, follow these guidelines:

Patient preparation
- Prepare the patient and his family for insertion, reinforcing explanations about the device, its purpose, and what to expect after insertion.
- Verify that an informed consent form has been signed.

- Continue close patient monitoring, including monitoring of continuous ECG, pulmonary artery and hemodynamic status, and intake and output.

Monitoring and aftercare

- Assess the patient's cardiovascular status, and monitor blood pressure and hemodynamic parameters, including cardiac output and cardiac index, ECG, and peripheral pulses.
- Inspect the incision and dressing at least every hour initially and then every 2 to 4 hours, as indicated by the patient's condition.
- Monitor urine output hourly, and maintain I.V. fluid therapy, as ordered. Watch for signs of fluid overload or decreasing urine output.
- Assess chest tube drainage and function frequently. Notify the practitioner if drainage is greater than 150 ml over 2 hours. Auscultate lungs for evidence of abnormal breath sounds or adventitious sounds. Evaluate oxygen saturation or mixed venous oxygen saturation levels, and administer oxygen, as needed and ordered.
- Obtain hemoglobin levels, hematocrit, and coagulation studies, as ordered. Administer blood component therapy, as indicated and ordered.
- Assess for signs and symptoms of bleeding.
- Administer antibiotics prophylactically, as ordered, to prevent infection.

PATIENT TEACHING

Before discharge after the insertion of a VAD, instruct the patient to:
- immediately report redness, swelling, or drainage at the incision site; chest pain; or fever
- immediately notify the practitioner of any signs or symptoms of heart failure (weight gain, dyspnea, edema)
- follow the prescribed medication regimen and report adverse effects
- follow his prescribed diet, especially sodium and fat restrictions
- maintain a balance between activity and rest
- follow his exercise or rehabilitation program, if prescribed
- comply with the laboratory schedule for monitoring International Normalized Ratio if the patient is receiving warfarin (Coumadin).

PART 5

Reviewing rhythm strips

16

PRACTICE STRIPS

Sharpening interpretation skills

Use these sample rhythm strips as a practical way to sharpen your electrocardiogram (ECG) interpretation skills. Record the rhythm, rates, and waveform characteristics in the blank spaces provided, and then compare your findings with the answers beginning on page 235.

1.

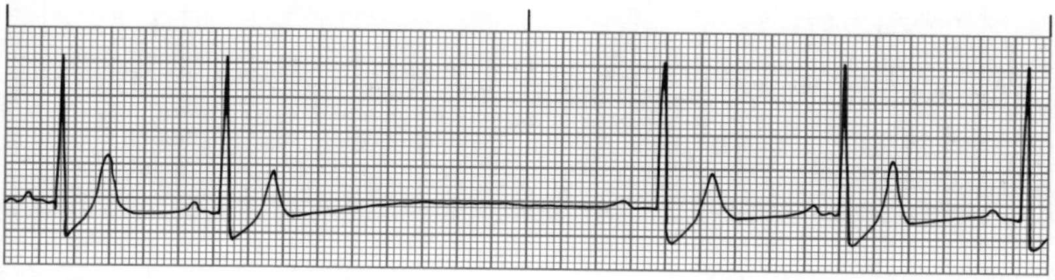

Atrial rhythm: ______________________________

Ventricular rhythm: ______________________________

Atrial rate: ______________________________

Ventricular rate: ______________________________

P wave: ______________________________

PR interval: ______________________________

QRS complex: ______________________________

T wave: ______________________________

QT interval: ______________________________

Other: ______________________________

Interpretation: ______________________________

2.

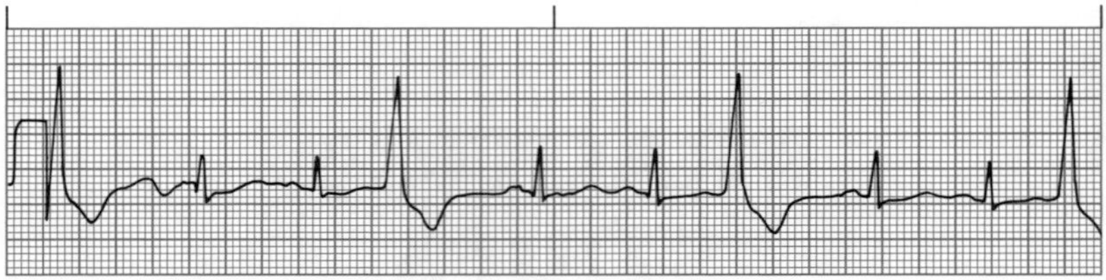

Atrial rhythm: _____

Ventricular rhythm: _____

Atrial rate: _____

Ventricular rate: _____

P wave: _____

PR interval: _____

QRS complex: _____

T wave: _____

QT interval: _____

Other: _____

Interpretation: _____

3.

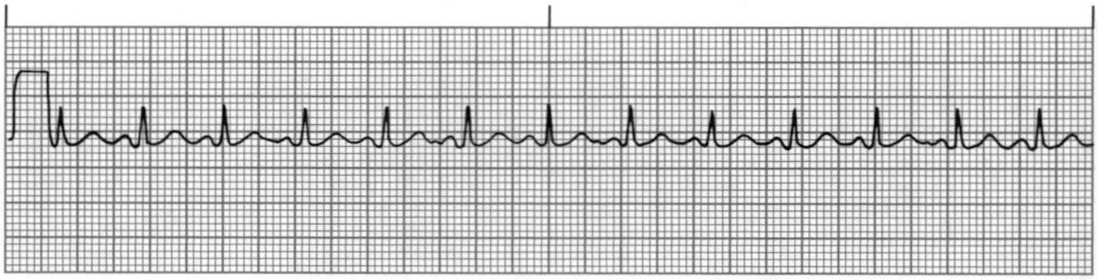

Atrial rhythm: _____

Ventricular rhythm: _____

Atrial rate: _____

Ventricular rate: _____

P wave: _____

PR interval: _____

QRS complex: _____

T wave: _____

QT interval: _____

Other: _____

Interpretation: _____

4.

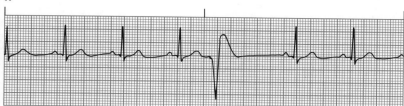

Atrial rhythm: _____

Ventricular rhythm:_____

Atrial rate: _____

Ventricular rate:_____

P wave: _____

PR interval: _____

QRS complex:_____

T wave: _____

QT interval: _____

Other:_____

Interpretation: _____

5.

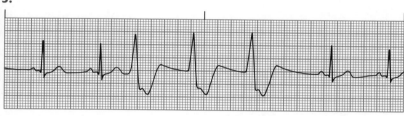

Atrial rhythm: _____

Ventricular rhythm:_____

Atrial rate: _____

Ventricular rate:_____

P wave: _____

PR interval: _____

QRS complex:_____

T wave: _____

QT interval: _____

Other:_____

Interpretation: _____

6.

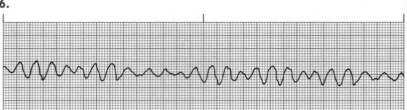

Atrial rhythm: _____
Ventricular rhythm: _____
Atrial rate: _____
Ventricular rate: _____
P wave: _____
PR interval: _____
QRS complex: _____
T wave: _____
QT interval: _____
Other: _____
Interpretation: _____

7.

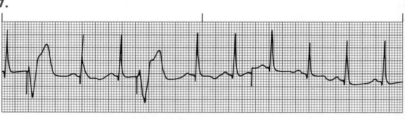

Atrial rhythm: _____
Ventricular rhythm: _____
Atrial rate: _____
Ventricular rate: _____
P wave: _____
PR interval: _____
QRS complex: _____
T wave: _____
QT interval: _____
Other: _____
Interpretation: _____

8.

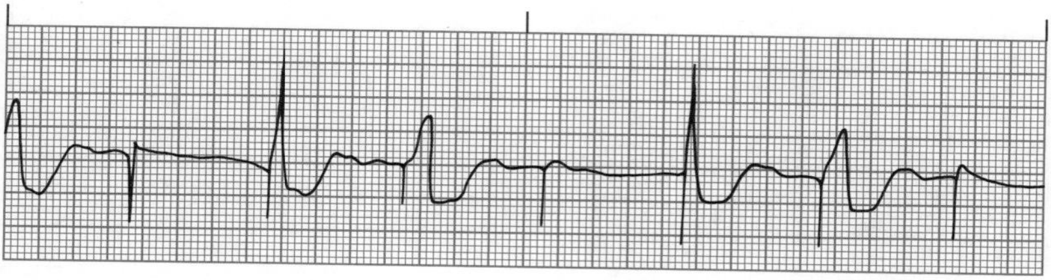

Atrial rhythm: _____

Ventricular rhythm:_____

Atrial rate: _____

Ventricular rate:_____

P wave: _____

PR interval: _____

QRS complex:_____

T wave: _____

QT interval: _____

Other:_____

Interpretation: _____

9.

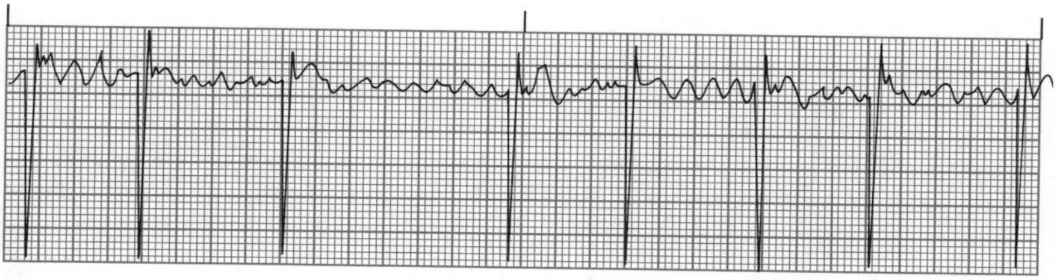

Atrial rhythm: _____

Ventricular rhythm:_____

Atrial rate: _____

Ventricular rate:_____

P wave: _____

PR interval: _____

QRS complex:_____

T wave: _____

QT interval: _____

Other:_____

Interpretation: _____

10.

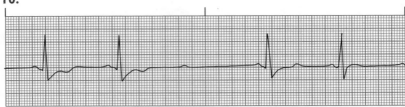

Atrial rhythm: _____

Ventricular rhythm:_____

Atrial rate: _____

Ventricular rate:_____

P wave: _____

PR interval: _____

QRS complex:_____

T wave: _____

QT interval: _____

Other:_____

Interpretation: _____

11.

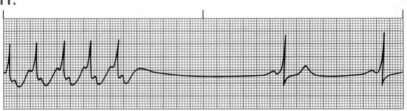

Atrial rhythm: _____

Ventricular rhythm:_____

Atrial rate: _____

Ventricular rate:_____

P wave: _____

PR interval: _____

QRS complex:_____

T wave: _____

QT interval: _____

Other:_____

Interpretation: _____

12.

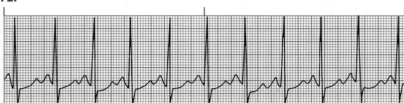

Atrial rhythm: _____

Ventricular rhythm:_____

Atrial rate: _____

Ventricular rate:_____

P wave: _____

PR interval: _____

QRS complex:_____

T wave: _____

QT interval: _____

Other:_____

Interpretation: _____

13.

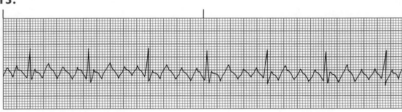

Atrial rhythm: _____

Ventricular rhythm:_____

Atrial rate: _____

Ventricular rate:_____

P wave: _____

PR interval: _____

QRS complex: _____

T wave: _____

QT interval: _____

Other:_____

Interpretation: _____

14.

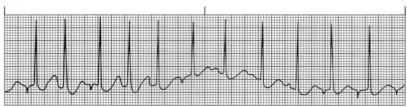

Atrial rhythm: _____

Ventricular rhythm: _____

Atrial rate: _____

Ventricular rate: _____

P wave: _____

PR interval: _____

QRS complex: _____

T wave: _____

QT interval: _____

Other: _____

Interpretation: _____

15.

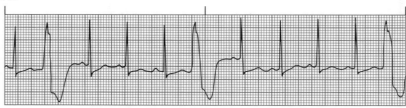

Atrial rhythm: _____

Ventricular rhythm: _____

Atrial rate: _____

Ventricular rate: _____

P wave: _____

PR interval: _____

QRS complex: _____

T wave: _____

QT interval: _____

Other: _____

Interpretation: _____

16.

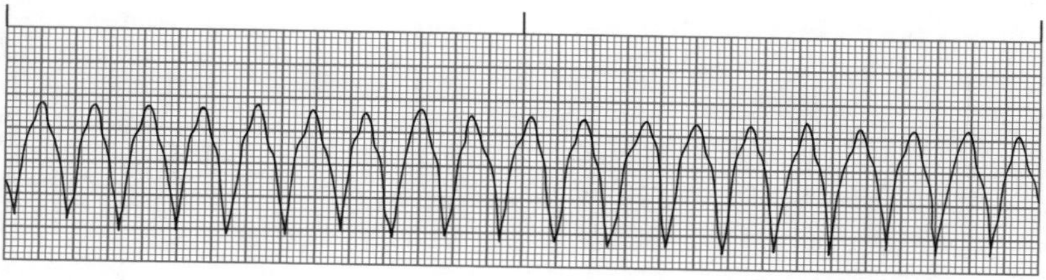

Atrial rhythm: _____
Ventricular rhythm:_____
Atrial rate: _____
Ventricular rate:_____
P wave: _____
PR interval: _____
QRS complex:_____
T wave: _____
QT interval: _____
Other:_____
Interpretation: _____

17.

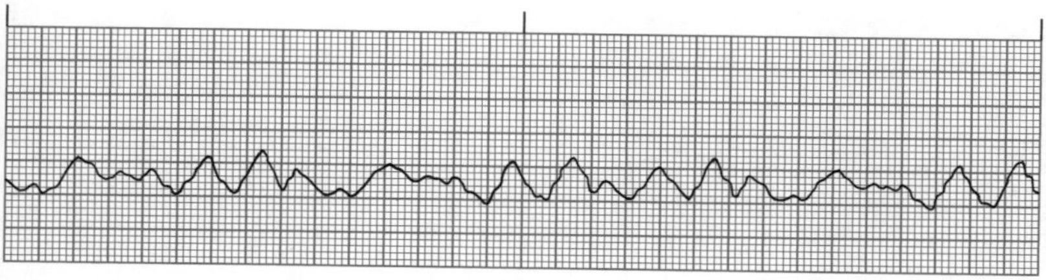

Atrial rhythm: _____
Ventricular rhythm:_____
Atrial rate: _____
Ventricular rate:_____
P wave: _____
PR interval: _____
QRS complex:_____
T wave: _____
QT interval: _____
Other:_____
Interpretation: _____

18.

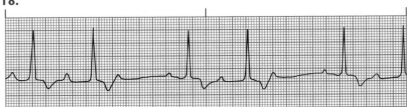

Atrial rhythm: _____

Ventricular rhythm:_____

Atrial rate: _____

Ventricular rate:_____

P wave: _____

PR interval: _____

QRS complex:_____

T wave: _____

QT interval: _____

Other:_____

Interpretation: _____

19.

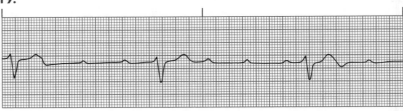

Atrial rhythm: _____

Ventricular rhythm:_____

Atrial rate: _____

Ventricular rate:_____

P wave: _____

PR interval: _____

QRS complex:_____

T wave: _____

QT interval: _____

Other:_____

Interpretation: _____

20.

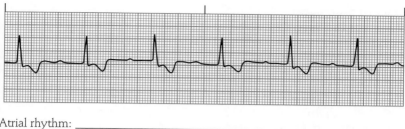

Atrial rhythm: _____

Ventricular rhythm:_____

Atrial rate: _____

Ventricular rate:_____

P wave: _____

PR interval: _____

QRS complex:_____

T wave: _____

QT interval: _____

Other:_____

Interpretation: _____

Sharpening interpretation skills: Answers

1.

Atrial rhythm: Regular, except for missing PQRST complex

Ventricular rhythm: Regular, except for missing PQRST complex

Atrial rate: 50 beats/minute; underlying rate 60 beats/minute

Ventricular rate: 50 beats/minute

P wave: Normal size and configuration; absent during pause

PR interval: 0.20 second

QRS complex: 0.08 second

T wave: Normal configuration; absent during pause

QT interval: 0.40 second

Other: None

Interpretation: Sinus arrest

2.

Atrial rhythm: Irregular
Ventricular rhythm: Irregular
Atrial rate: 60 beats/minute; underlying rate 88 beats/minute
Ventricular rate: 90 beats/minute
P wave: None with premature ventricular contractions (PVCs); present with QRS complexes
PR interval: 0.16 second
QRS complex: Underlying rate 0.08 second; 0.16 second with PVCs
T wave: Normal configuration; opposite direction with PVCs
QT interval: 0.42 second
Other: None
Interpretation: Normal sinus rhythm with trigeminal PVCs

3.

Atrial rhythm: Regular
Ventricular rhythm: Regular
Atrial rate: 125 beats/minute
Ventricular rate: 125 beats/minute
P wave: Normal size and configuration
PR interval: 0.14 second
QRS complex: 0.08 second
T wave: Normal configuration
QT interval: 0.32 second
Other: None
Interpretation: Sinus tachycardia

4.

Atrial rhythm: Irregular
Ventricular rhythm: Irregular
Atrial rate: 60 beats/minute; underlying rate 71 beats/minute
Ventricular rate: 70 beats/minute
P wave: None with PVC; present with QRS complexes
PR interval: 0.16 second
QRS complex: 0.08 second; 0.14 second with PVC
T wave: Normal configuration
QT interval: 0.40 second
Other: None
Interpretation: Normal sinus rhythm with PVC

5.

Atrial rhythm: Irregular
Ventricular rhythm: Irregular
Atrial rate: 40 beats/minute; underlying rate 70 beats/minute

Ventricular rate: 70 beats/minute
P wave: None with PVCs; present with QRS complexes
PR interval: 0.16 second
QRS complex: 0.08 second; 0.16 second with PVCs
T wave: Normal configuration
QT interval: 0.40 second
Other: None
Interpretation: Normal sinus rhythm with run of PVCs

6.

Atrial rhythm: Absent
Ventricular rhythm: Chaotic
Atrial rate: Absent
Ventricular rate: Undetermined
P wave: Absent
PR interval: Unmeasurable
QRS complex: Indiscernible
T wave: Indiscernible
QT interval: Not applicable
Other: None
Interpretation: Ventricular fibrillation

7.

Atrial rhythm: Regular
Ventricular rhythm: Regular
Atrial rate: 90 beats/minute; underlying rate 107 beats/minute
Ventricular rate: 110 beats/minute
P wave: Present in normal QRS complexes
PR interval: 0.16 second
QRS complex: 0.08 second
T wave: Normal configuration
QT interval: 0.32 second
Other: Random pacemaker spikes
Interpretation: Sinus tachycardia with pacemaker failure to sense

8.

Atrial rhythm: Unmeasurable
Ventricular rhythm: Regular
Atrial rate: Unmeasurable
Ventricular rate: Paced rate 40 beats/minute; pacer fires at 75 beats/minute
P wave: Absent
PR interval: Unmeasurable
QRS complex: Unmeasurable
T wave: Unidentifiable

QT interval: Unmeasurable
Other: None
Interpretation: Paced rhythm with failure to capture

9.

Atrial rhythm: Irregular
Ventricular rhythm: Irregular
Atrial rate: Indiscernible
Ventricular rate: 60 beats/minute
P wave: Absent; fine fibrillation waves present
PR interval: Indiscernible
QRS complex: 0.08 second
T wave: Indiscernible
QT interval: Unmeasurable
Other: None
Interpretation: Atrial fibrillation

10.

Atrial rhythm: Regular
Ventricular rhythm: Irregular
Atrial rate: 50 beats/minute
Ventricular rate: 30 beats/minute
P wave: Normal; some not followed by QRS complexes
PR interval: 0.16 second and constant for conducted impulses
QRS complex: 0.08 second
T wave: Normal configuration; absent if QRS complexes are absent
QT interval: 0.40 second
Other: None
Interpretation: Type II second-degree atrioventricular (AV) block

11.

Atrial rhythm: Irregular
Ventricular rhythm: Irregular
Atrial rate: 60 beats/minute
Ventricular rate: 70 beats/minute
P wave: Rate and configuration varies
PR interval: Varies with rhythm
QRS complex: 0.10 second
T wave: Configuration varies
QT interval: Configuration varies
Other: None
Interpretation: Sick sinus syndrome

12.

Atrial rhythm: Regular
Ventricular rhythm: Regular
Atrial rate: 110 beats/minute
Ventricular rate: 110 beats/minute
P wave: Normal size and configuration
PR interval: 0.16 second
QRS complex: 0.10 second
T wave: Normal configuration
QT interval: 0.36 second
Other: None
Interpretation: Sinus tachycardia

13.

Atrial rhythm: Regular
Ventricular rhythm: Regular
Atrial rate: 270 beats/minute
Ventricular rate: 70 beats/minute
P wave: Saw-tooth edged
PR interval: Unmeasurable
QRS complex: 0.10 second
T wave: Unidentifiable
QT interval: Unidentifiable
Other: None
Interpretation: Atrial flutter (4:1 block)

14.

Atrial rhythm: Irregular
Ventricular rhythm: Irregular
Atrial rate: About 150 beats/minute
Ventricular rate: About 150 beats/minute
P wave: Size and configuration vary
PR interval: Rate varies
QRS complex: 0.08 second
T wave: Inverted
QT interval: 0.22 second
Other: None
Interpretation: Multifocal atrial tachycardia

15.

Atrial rhythm: Irregular
Ventricular rhythm: Irregular
Atrial rate: 105 beats/minute

Ventricular rate: 105 beats/minute
P wave: Normal size and configuration, except during premature beat
PR interval: 0.16 second; unmeasurable for premature beat
QRS complex: 0.06 second
T wave: Normal configuration
QT interval: 0.36 second
Other: None
Interpretation: Sinus tachycardia with PVCs

16.
Atrial rhythm: Unmeasurable
Ventricular rhythm: Regular
Atrial rate: Unmeasurable
Ventricular rate: 187 beats/minute
P wave: Absent
PR interval: Unmeasurable
QRS complex: 0.18 second; wide and bizarre
T wave: Opposite direction of QRS complex
QT interval: Unmeasurable
Other: None
Interpretation: Ventricular tachycardia (monomorphic)

17.
Atrial rhythm: Absent
Ventricular rhythm: Chaotic
Atrial rate: Absent
Ventricular rate: Unmeasurable
P wave: Absent
PR interval: Absent
QRS complex: Indiscernible
T wave: Indiscernible
QT interval: Absent
Other: None
Interpretation: Ventricular fibrillation

18.
Atrial rhythm: Regular
Ventricular rhythm: Irregular
Atrial rate: 75 beats/minute
Ventricular rate: 50 beats/minute
P wave: Normal size and configuration
PR interval: Lengthens with each cycle until dropped

QRS complex: 0.06 second
T wave: Normal configuration
QT interval: 0.38 second
Other: None
Interpretation: Type I (Mobitz I or Wenckebach) second-degree AV block

19.

Atrial rhythm: Regular
Ventricular rhythm: Regular
Atrial rate: 90 beats/minute
Ventricular rate: 30 beats/minute
P wave: Normal size and configuration, except when hidden within T wave
PR interval: Rate varies
QRS complex: 0.16 second
T wave: Normal configuration
QT interval: 0.56 second
Other: None
Interpretation: Third-degree AV block

20.

Atrial rhythm: Regular
Ventricular rhythm: Regular
Atrial rate: 60 beats/minute
Ventricular rate: 60 beats/minute
P wave: Normal size and configuration
PR interval: 0.36 second
QRS complex: 0.08 second
T wave: Normal configuration
QT interval: 0.40 second
Other: None
Interpretation: Normal sinus rhythm with first-degree AV block

ECG challenge: Differentiating rhythm strips

Differentiating ECG rhythm strips can often be daunting, especially when waveform patterns appear strikingly similar. These pairs of rhythm strips are among the most challenging to interpret. Test your knowledge and skill by correctly identifying each rhythm strip; answers begin on page 245.

1.
Rhythm strip A

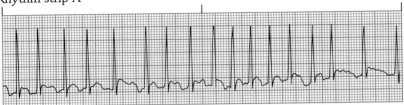

Rhythm strip A is:_____

Rhythm strip B

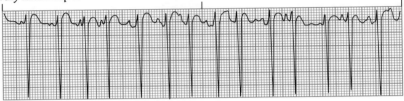

Rhythm strip B is:_____

2.
Rhythm strip A

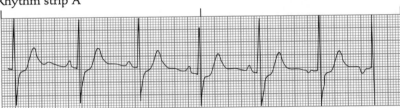

Rhythm strip A is:_____

Rhythm strip B

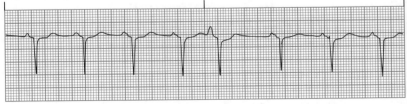

Rhythm strip B is:_____

3.

Rhythm strip A

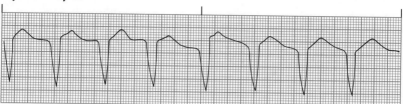

Rhythm strip A is: _____

Rhythm strip B

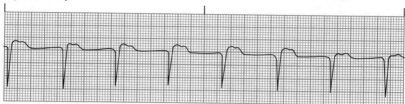

Rhythm strip B is: _____

4.

Rhythm strip A

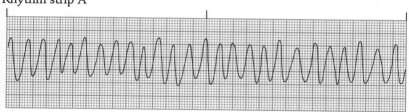

Rhythm strip A is: _____

Rhythm strip B

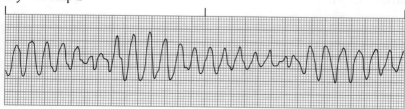

Rhythm strip B is: _____

5.
Rhythm strip A

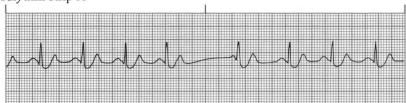

Rhythm strip A is: _____ :

Rhythm strip B

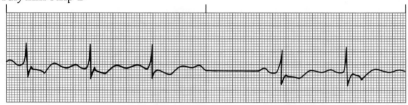

Rhythm strip B is: _____

6.
Rhythm strip A

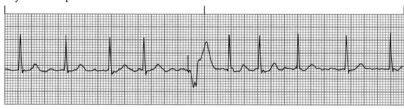

Rhythm strip A is:_____

Rhythm strip B

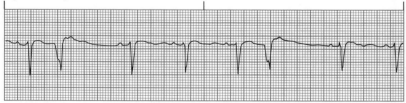

Rhythm strip B is: _____

ECG challenge: Differentiating rhythm strips—Answers

1.

Rhythm strip A: Atrial fibrillation
Rhythm strip B: Multifocal atrial tachycardia (MAT)
To help you decide whether a rhythm is atrial fibrillation or the similar MAT, focus on the presence of P waves as well as the atrial and ventricular rhythms. You may find it helpful to look at a longer (greater than 6 seconds) rhythm strip.

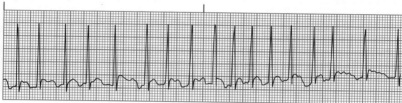

Atrial fibrillation
- Carefully look for discernible P waves before each QRS complex.
- If you can't clearly identify P waves, if fibrillatory waves appear in place of P waves, and if the rhythm is irregular, then the rhythm is probably atrial fibrillation.
- Carefully look at the rhythm, focusing on the R-R intervals. Remember that one of the hallmarks of atrial fibrillation is an irregularly irregular rhythm.

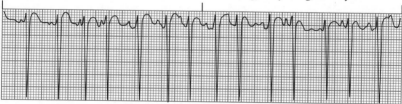

Multifocal atrial tachycardia
- P waves are present in MAT. Keep in mind, however, that the shape of the P waves will vary, with at least three different P wave shapes visible in a single rhythm strip.
- You should be able to see most, if not all, of the various P wave shapes repeat.
- Although the atrial and ventricular rhythms are irregular, the irregularity generally isn't as pronounced as in atrial fibrillation.

2.

Rhythm strip A: Wandering pacemaker
Rhythm strip B: Premature atrial contraction (PAC)

Because PACs are commonly encountered, it's possible to mistake wandering pacemaker for PACs unless the rhythm strip is carefully examined. In such cases, you may find it helpful to look at a longer (greater than 6 seconds) rhythm strip.

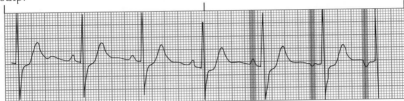

Wandering pacemaker

● Carefully examine the P waves. You must be able to identify at least three different shapes of P waves (see shaded areas above) in wandering pacemaker.
● Atrial rhythm varies slightly, with an irregular P-P interval. Ventricular rhythm also varies slightly, with an irregular R-R interval. These slight variations in rhythm result from the changing site of impulse formation.

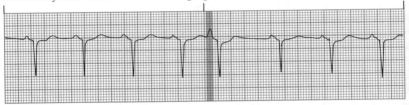

Premature atrial contraction

● The PAC occurs earlier than the sinus P wave, with an abnormal configuration when compared with a sinus P wave (see shaded area above). It's possible (but rare) to see multifocal PACs that originate from multiple ectopic pacemaker sites in the atria. In this setting, the P waves have different shapes.
● With the exception of the irregular atrial and ventricular rhythms that result from the PAC, the underlying rhythm is usually regular.

3.

Rhythm strip A: Accelerated idioventricular rhythm
Rhythm strip B: Accelerated junctional rhythm

Accelerated idioventricular rhythm and accelerated junctional rhythm appear similar, but have different causes. To distinguish between the two, closely examine the duration of the QRS complex and then look for P waves.

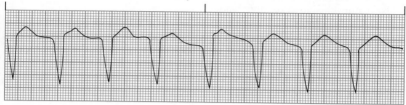

Accelerated idioventricular rhythm

- The QRS duration will be greater than 0.12 second.
- The QRS complex will have a wide and bizarre configuration.
- P waves are usually absent.
- The ventricular rate is generally between 40 and 100 beats/minute.

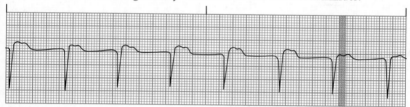

Accelerated junctional rhythm

- The QRS duration and configuration are usually normal.
- Inverted P waves generally occur before or after the QRS complex (see shaded area above). However, remember that P waves also may be buried within QRS complexes.
- The ventricular rate is typically between 60 and 100 beats/minute.

4.

Rhythm strip A: Ventricular flutter
Rhythm strip B: Torsades de pointes

Ventricular flutter, although rarely recognized, results from the rapid, regular, repetitive beating of the ventricles. It's produced by a single ventricular focus firing at a rapid rate of 250 to 350 beats/minute. The hallmark of this arrhythmia is its smooth sine-wave appearance.

Torsades de pointes is a variant form of ventricular tachycardia, with a rapid ventricular rate that varies between 150 and 300 beats/minute. It's characterized by QRS complexes that gradually change back and forth, with the amplitude of each successive complex gradually increasing, and then decreasing. This results in an overall outline of the rhythm commonly described as *spindle-shaped*.

The illustrations shown here highlight key differences in the two arrhythmias.

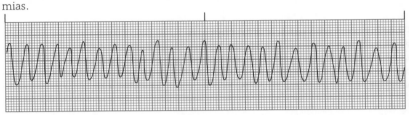

Ventricular flutter
- Smooth sine-wave appearance

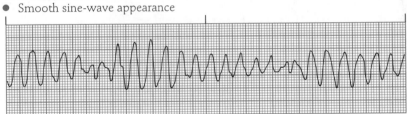

Torsades de pointes
- Spindle-shaped appearance

5.

Rhythm strip A: Nonconducted PAC
Rhythm strip B: Type II second-degree AV block

An isolated P wave that doesn't conduct through to the ventricle (P wave without a QRS complex following it; see shaded areas in both illustrations below) may occur with either a nonconducted PAC or type II second-degree AV block. To differentiate the two, look for constancy of the P-P interval. Be aware that mistakenly identifying AV block as nonconducted PACs may have serious consequences. The latter is generally benign, whereas the former can be life-threatening.

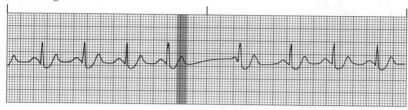

Nonconducted PAC
● If the P-P interval (including the extra P wave) isn't constant, it's a nonconducted PAC.

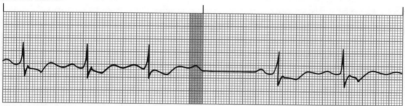

Type II second-degree AV block
● If the P-P interval is constant, including the extra P wave, it's type II second-degree AV block.

6.

Rhythm strip A: Intermittent ventricular pacing
Rhythm strip B: Premature ventricular contraction

Knowing whether your patient has an artificial pacemaker will help you avoid mistaking a ventricular paced beat for a PVC. If your facility uses a monitoring system that eliminates artifact, make sure the monitor is set up correctly for a patient with a pacemaker. Otherwise, the pacemaker spikes may be eliminated as well.

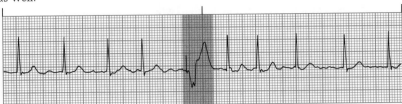

Intermittent ventricular pacing

● The paced ventricular complex will have a pacemaker spike preceding it (see shaded area above). You may need to look in different leads for a bipolar pacemaker spike because it's small and may be difficult to see.
● The paced ventricular complex of a properly functioning pacemaker won't occur early or prematurely. It will occur only when the patient's own ventricular rate falls below the rate set for the pacemaker.

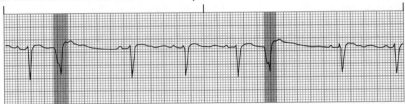

Premature ventricular contraction

● PVCs will occur prematurely and won't have pacemaker spikes preceding them (see shaded areas above).

RAPID REFERENCE TO MAJOR ARRHYTHMIAS

ACLS ALGORITHMS

CARDIAC DRUG OVERVIEW

SELECTED REFERENCES

INDEX

———◆———

RAPID REFERENCE TO MAJOR ARRHYTHMIAS

SINUS ARRHYTHMIA

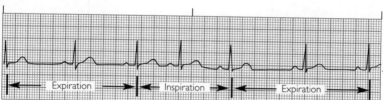

FEATURES
◆ Rhythm irregular; varies with respiratory cycle
◆ P-P and R-R intervals shorter during inspiration, longer during expiration
◆ Normal P wave preceding each QRS complex

SINUS BRADYCARDIA

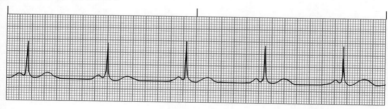

FEATURES
◆ Rhythm regular
◆ Atrial and ventricular rates < 60 beats/minute
◆ Normal P wave preceding each QRS complex
◆ Normal QRS complex
◆ QT interval may be prolonged

Sinus tachycardia

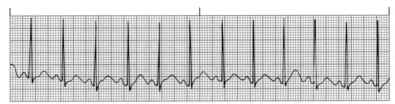

Features
◆ Rhythm regular
◆ Atrial and ventricular rates >100 beats/minute
◆ Normal P wave preceding each QRS complex
◆ Normal QRS complex
◆ QT interval commonly shortened

Sinus arrest

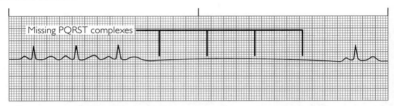

Features
◆ Rhythm normal, except for missing PQRST complexes
◆ P wave is periodically absent with entire PQRST complexes missing; when present, normal P wave precedes each QRS complex

Premature atrial contractions (PACs)

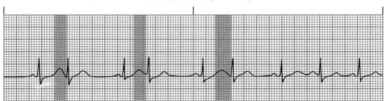

Features
◆ Premature, abnormal P waves (differ in configuration from normal P waves)
◆ QRS complexes after P waves, except in blocked PACs
◆ P wave often buried or identified in preceding T wave

ATRIAL TACHYCARDIA

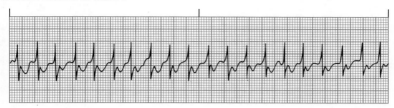

FEATURES
◆ Rhythm regular if block is constant; irregular if not
◆ Rate 150 to 250 beats/minute
◆ P waves regular but hidden in preceding T wave; precede QRS complexes

ATRIAL FLUTTER

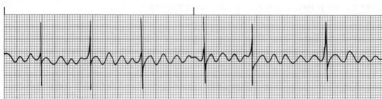

FEATURES
◆ Atrial rhythm regular; ventricular rhythm variable
◆ Atrial rate 250 to 400 beats/minute; ventricular rate depends on degree of atrioventricular (AV) block
◆ Sawtooth P-wave configuration (flutter waves)

ATRIAL FIBRILLATION

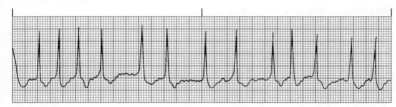

FEATURES
◆ Atrial and ventricular rhythms grossly irregular
◆ Atrial rate > 400 beats/minute; ventricular rate varies
◆ No P waves; replaced by fine fibrillatory waves

Wandering pacemaker

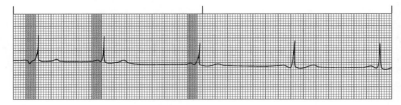

FEATURES
◆ Rhythm irregular
◆ PR interval varies
◆ P waves change in configuration, indicating origin in sinoatrial node, atria, or AV junction (*Hallmark:* At least three different P wave configurations)

PREMATURE JUNCTIONAL CONTRACTIONS (PJCS)

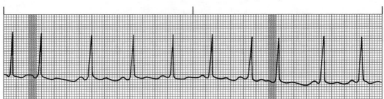

FEATURES
◆ Rhythm irregular during PJCs
◆ P waves before, hidden in, or after QRS complexes; inverted if visible
◆ PR interval < 0.12 second, if P wave precedes QRS complex
◆ QRS configuration and duration normal

JUNCTIONAL ESCAPE RHYTHM

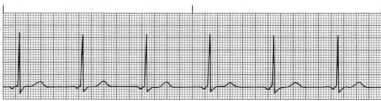

FEATURES
◆ Rhythm regular
◆ Rate 40 to 60 beats/minute
◆ P waves before, hidden in, or after QRS complexes; inverted if visible
◆ PR interval < 0.12 second (measurable only if P wave appears before QRS complex)

JUNCTIONAL TACHYCARDIA

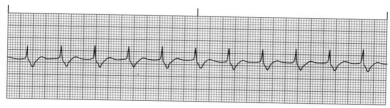

FEATURES

◆ Rhythm regular
◆ Rate 100 to 200 beats/minute
◆ P waves before, hidden in, or after QRS complexes; inverted if visible

PREMATURE VENTRICULAR CONTRACTIONS (PVCs)

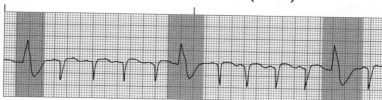

FEATURES

◆ Underlying rhythm regular; P wave absent with PVCs
◆ Ventricular rhythm irregular during PVC
◆ QRS premature, usually followed by compensatory pause
◆ QRS complex wide and bizarre, duration > 0.12 second
◆ Premature QRS complexes occurring singly, in pairs, or in threes; possibly unifocal or multi-formed
◆ Most ominous when clustered, multiformed, and with R wave on T pattern

VENTRICULAR TACHYCARDIA

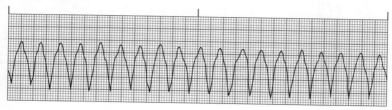

FEATURES

◆ Atrial rhythm can't be determined; ventricular rhythm usually regular
◆ Ventricular rate 100 to 250 beats/minute
◆ QRS complexes wide and bizarre; duration > 0.12 second
◆ P waves indiscernible

VENTRICULAR FIBRILLATION

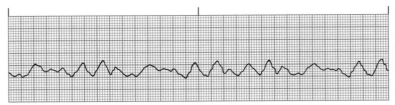

FEATURES
◆ Atrial rhythm can't be determined
◆ Ventricular rhythm has no pattern, just chaotic fibrillatory waves
◆ Atrial and ventricular rates can't be determined
◆ No discernible P waves, QRS complexes, or T waves

ASYSTOLE

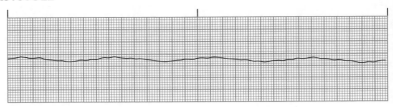

FEATURES
◆ No atrial or ventricular rhythm or rate
◆ No discernible P waves, QRS complexes, or T waves

FIRST-DEGREE AV BLOCK

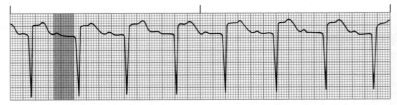

FEATURES
◆ Rhythm regular
◆ PR interval > 0.20 second and constant
◆ P wave preceding each QRS complex; QRS complex normal

Type I second-degree AV block (Mobitz Type I, Wenckebach)

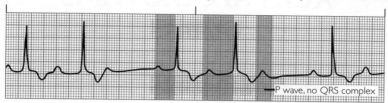

— P wave, no QRS complex

FEATURES
◆ Atrial rhythm regular
◆ Ventricular rhythm irregular
◆ Atrial rate exceeds ventricular rate
◆ PR interval progressively longer with each cycle until a P wave appears without a QRS complex (dropped beat)

Type II second-degree AV block (Mobitz Type II)

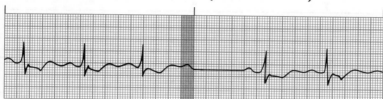

FEATURES
◆ Atrial rhythm regular
◆ Ventricular rhythm possibly irregular, varying with degree of block
◆ P waves normal size and configuration; some not followed by QRS complex
◆ PR interval is constant for conducted beats
◆ QRS complexes periodically absent

Third-degree AV block (complete heart block)

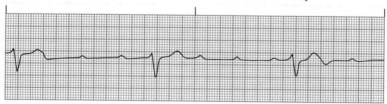

FEATURES
◆ Atrial and ventricular rhythms regular
◆ Ventricular rate is 40 to 60 beats/minute (AV node origin); < 40 beats/minute (Purkinje system origin)
◆ No relationship between P waves and QRS complexes
◆ QRS complex normal (originating in AV node) or wide and bizarre (originating in Purkinje system)

ACLS ALGORITHMS

PULSELESS ARREST

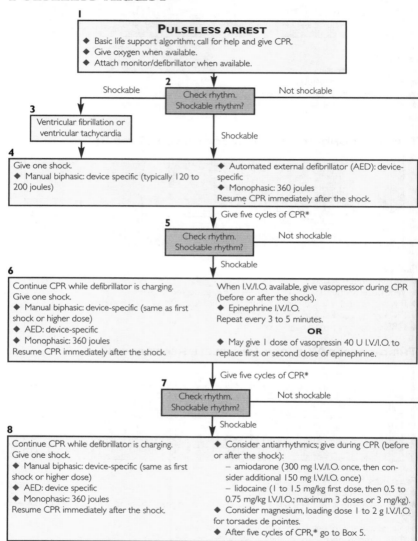

1

PULSELESS ARREST
- ◆ Basic life support algorithm; call for help and give CPR.
- ◆ Give oxygen when available.
- ◆ Attach monitor/defibrillator when available.

Shockable ⟶ **2** Check rhythm. Shockable rhythm? ⟵ Not shockable

3
Ventricular fibrillation or ventricular tachycardia

Shockable

4
Give one shock.
- ◆ Manual biphasic: device specific (typically 120 to 200 joules)

- ◆ Automated external defibrillator (AED): device-specific
- ◆ Monophasic: 360 joules
Resume CPR immediately after the shock.

Give five cycles of CPR*

5 Check rhythm. Shockable rhythm? ⟵ Not shockable

Shockable

6
Continue CPR while defibrillator is charging. Give one shock.
- ◆ Manual biphasic: device-specific (same as first shock or higher dose)
- ◆ AED: device-specific
- ◆ Monophasic: 360 joules
Resume CPR immediately after the shock.

When I.V./I.O. available, give vasopressor during CPR (before or after the shock).
- ◆ Epinephrine I.V./I.O.
Repeat every 3 to 5 minutes.
OR
- ◆ May give 1 dose of vasopressin 40 U I.V./I.O. to replace first or second dose of epinephrine.

Give five cycles of CPR*

7 Check rhythm. Shockable rhythm? ⟵ Not shockable

Shockable

8
Continue CPR while defibrillator is charging. Give one shock.
- ◆ Manual biphasic: device-specific (same as first shock or higher dose)
- ◆ AED: device specific
- ◆ Monophasic: 360 joules
Resume CPR immediately after the shock.

- ◆ Consider antiarrhythmics; give during CPR (before or after the shock):
  – amiodarone (300 mg I.V./I.O. once, then consider additional 150 mg I.V./I.O. once)
  – lidocaine (1 to 1.5 mg/kg first dose, then 0.5 to 0.75 mg/kg I.V./I.O.; maximum 3 doses or 3 mg/kg).
- ◆ Consider magnesium, loading dose 1 to 2 g I.V./I.O. for torsades de pointes.
- ◆ After five cycles of CPR,* go to Box 5.

* After an advanced airway is placed, rescuers no longer deliver "cycles" of CPR. Give continuous chest compressions without pauses for breaths. Give 8 to 10 breaths/minute. Check rhythm every 2 minutes.

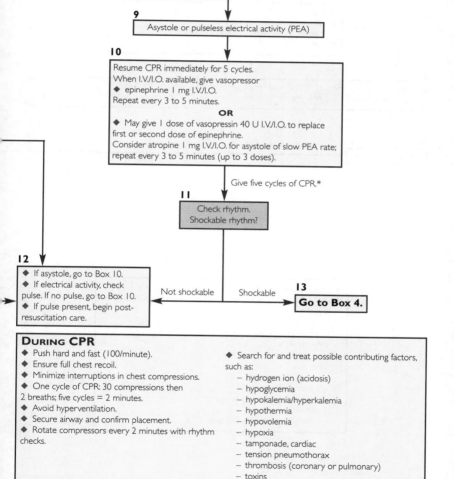

9

Asystole or pulseless electrical activity (PEA)

10

Resume CPR immediately for 5 cycles.
When I.V./I.O. available, give vasopressor
◆ epinephrine 1 mg I.V./I.O.
Repeat every 3 to 5 minutes.

OR

◆ May give 1 dose of vasopressin 40 U I.V./I.O. to replace
first or second dose of epinephrine.
Consider atropine 1 mg I.V./I.O. for asystole of slow PEA rate;
repeat every 3 to 5 minutes (up to 3 doses).

Give five cycles of CPR.*

11

Check rhythm.
Shockable rhythm?

12

◆ If asystole, go to Box 10.
◆ If electrical activity, check
pulse. If no pulse, go to Box 10.
◆ If pulse present, begin post-
resuscitation care.

Not shockable

Shockable

13

Go to Box 4.

DURING CPR

◆ Push hard and fast (100/minute).
◆ Ensure full chest recoil.
◆ Minimize interruptions in chest compressions.
◆ One cycle of CPR: 30 compressions then
2 breaths; five cycles = 2 minutes.
◆ Avoid hyperventilation.
◆ Secure airway and confirm placement.
◆ Rotate compressors every 2 minutes with rhythm
checks.

◆ Search for and treat possible contributing factors,
such as:
  – hydrogen ion (acidosis)
  – hypoglycemia
  – hypokalemia/hyperkalemia
  – hypothermia
  – hypovolemia
  – hypoxia
  – tamponade, cardiac
  – tension pneumothorax
  – thrombosis (coronary or pulmonary)
  – toxins
  – trauma.

BRADYCARDIA

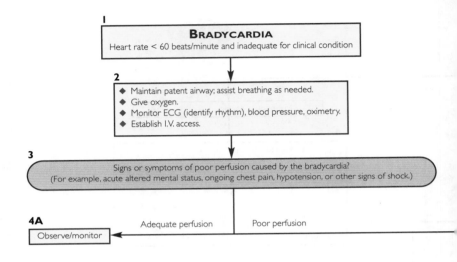

1

BRADYCARDIA
Heart rate < 60 beats/minute and inadequate for clinical condition

2
- ◆ Maintain patent airway; assist breathing as needed.
- ◆ Give oxygen.
- ◆ Monitor ECG (identify rhythm), blood pressure, oximetry.
- ◆ Establish I.V. access.

3
Signs or symptoms of poor perfusion caused by the bradycardia?
(For example, acute altered mental status, ongoing chest pain, hypotension, or other signs of shock.)

4A
| Adequate perfusion | Poor perfusion |

Observe/monitor

- ◆ If pulseless arrest develops, go to Pulseless Arrest Algorithm.
- ◆ Search for and treat possible contributing factors, such as:
  - hydrogen ion (acidosis)
  - hypoglycemia
  - hypokalemia/hyperkalemia
  - hypothermia
  - hypovolemia
  - hypoxia
  - tamponade, cardiac
  - tension pneumothorax
  - thrombosis (coronary or pulmonary)
  - toxins
  - trauma (hypovolemia, increased ICP).

4

◆ Prepare for transcutaneous pacing; use without delay for high-degree block (type II second-degree block or third-degree atrioventricular block).
◆ Consider atropine 0.5 mg I.V. while awaiting pacer. May repeat to a total dose of 3 mg. If ineffective, begin pacing.
◆ Consider epinephrine (2 to 10 mcg/minute) or dopamine (2 to 10 mcg/kg/minute) infusion while awaiting pacer or if pacing ineffective.

5

◆ Prepare for transvenous pacing.
◆ Treat contributing causes.
◆ Consider expert consultation.

TACHYCARDIA

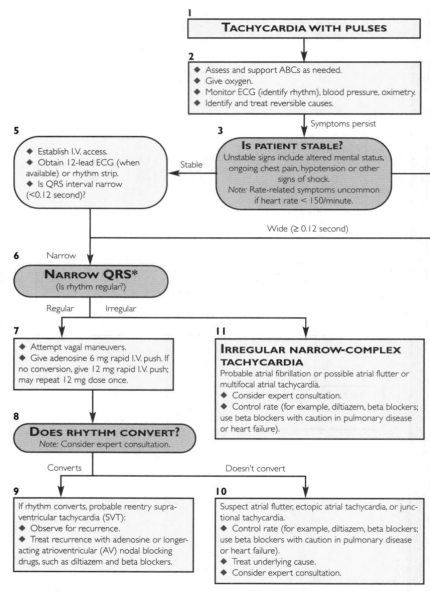

1

TACHYCARDIA WITH PULSES

2

- ◆ Assess and support ABCs as needed.
- ◆ Give oxygen.
- ◆ Monitor ECG (identify rhythm), blood pressure, oximetry.
- ◆ Identify and treat reversible causes.

Symptoms persist

5

- ◆ Establish I.V. access.
- ◆ Obtain 12-lead ECG (when available) or rhythm strip.
- ◆ Is QRS interval narrow (<0.12 second)?

Stable

3

IS PATIENT STABLE?
Unstable signs include altered mental status, ongoing chest pain, hypotension or other signs of shock.
Note: Rate-related symptoms uncommon if heart rate < 150/minute.

Wide (≥ 0.12 second)

6   Narrow

NARROW QRS*
(Is rhythm regular?)

Regular   Irregular

7

- ◆ Attempt vagal maneuvers.
- ◆ Give adenosine 6 mg rapid I.V. push. If no conversion, give 12 mg rapid I.V. push; may repeat 12 mg dose once.

11

IRREGULAR NARROW-COMPLEX TACHYCARDIA
Probable atrial fibrillation or possible atrial flutter or multifocal atrial tachycardia.
- ◆ Consider expert consultation.
- ◆ Control rate (for example, diltiazem, beta blockers; use beta blockers with caution in pulmonary disease or heart failure).

8

DOES RHYTHM CONVERT?
Note: Consider expert consultation.

Converts   Doesn't convert

9

If rhythm converts, probable reentry supraventricular tachycardia (SVT):
- ◆ Observe for recurrence.
- ◆ Treat recurrence with adenosine or longer-acting atrioventricular (AV) nodal blocking drugs, such as diltiazem and beta blockers.

10

Suspect atrial flutter, ectopic atrial tachycardia, or junctional tachycardia.
- ◆ Control rate (for example, diltiazem, beta blockers; use beta blockers with caution in pulmonary disease or heart failure).
- ◆ Treat underlying cause.
- ◆ Consider expert consultation.

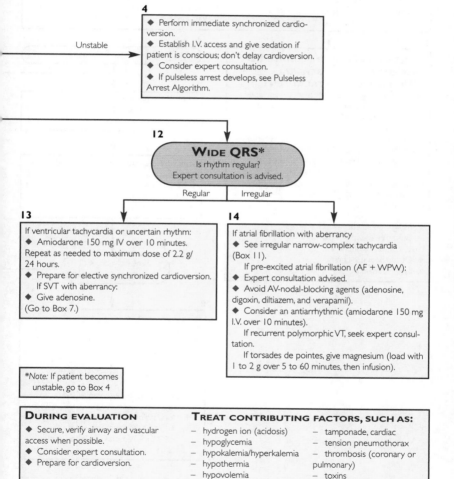

4
- ◆ Perform immediate synchronized cardio-version.
- ◆ Establish I.V. access and give sedation if patient is conscious; don't delay cardioversion.
- ◆ Consider expert consultation.
- ◆ If pulseless arrest develops, see Pulseless Arrest Algorithm.

Unstable

12

WIDE QRS*
Is rhythm regular?
Expert consultation is advised.

Regular | Irregular

13
If ventricular tachycardia or uncertain rhythm:
- ◆ Amiodarone 150 mg IV over 10 minutes. Repeat as needed to maximum dose of 2.2 g/ 24 hours.
- ◆ Prepare for elective synchronized cardioversion. If SVT with aberrancy:
- ◆ Give adenosine. (Go to Box 7.)

14
If atrial fibrillation with aberrancy
- ◆ See irregular narrow-complex tachycardia (Box 11).
  If pre-excited atrial fibrillation (AF + WPW):
- ◆ Expert consultation advised.
- ◆ Avoid AV-nodal-blocking agents (adenosine, digoxin, diltiazem, and verapamil).
- ◆ Consider an antiarrhythmic (amiodarone 150 mg I.V. over 10 minutes).
  If recurrent polymorphic VT, seek expert consultation.
  If torsades de pointes, give magnesium (load with 1 to 2 g over 5 to 60 minutes, then infusion).

*Note: If patient becomes unstable, go to Box 4

DURING EVALUATION
- ◆ Secure, verify airway and vascular access when possible.
- ◆ Consider expert consultation.
- ◆ Prepare for cardioversion.

TREAT CONTRIBUTING FACTORS, SUCH AS:
- – hydrogen ion (acidosis)
- – hypoglycemia
- – hypokalemia/hyperkalemia
- – hypothermia
- – hypovolemia
- – hypoxia
- – tamponade, cardiac
- – tension pneumothorax
- – thrombosis (coronary or pulmonary)
- – toxins
- – trauma (hypovolemia).

ACUTE CORONARY SYNDROME

1

CHEST DISCOMFORT SUGGESTIVE OF ISCHEMIA

2

EMS ASSESSMENT AND CARE AND HOSPITAL PREPARATION
- Monitor, support ABCs. Be prepared to provide CPR and defibrillation.
- Administer oxygen, aspirin, nitroglycerin, and morphine, if needed.

- If available, obtain 12-lead ECG; if ST elevation:
  – Notify receiving hospital with transmission or interpretation.
  – Begin fibrinolytic checklist.
- Hospital should mobilize resources to respond to ST-elevation myocardial infarction (STEMI).

3

IMMEDIATE ED ASSESSMENT (<10 MINUTE)
- Check vital signs; evaluate oxygen saturation.
- Establish I.V. access.
- Obtain/review 12-lead ECG.
- Perform brief, targeted history, physical examination.
- Obtain initial cardiac marker levels, initial electrolyte and coagulation studies.
- Review/complete fibrinolytic checklist; check contraindication.
- Obtain portable chest X-ray (<30 minute).

IMMEDIATE ED GENERAL TREATMENT
- Start oxygen at 4 L/minute; maintain 02 saturation > 90%
- 160 to 325 mg aspirin (if not given by EMS)
- Nitroglycerin sublingual, spray, or I.V.
- Morphine I.V. if pain not relieved by nitroglycerin

4

Review initial 12-lead ECG.

5

ST elevation or new or presumably new left bundle-branch block; strongly suspicious for injury STEMI

6

Start adjunctive treatment as indicated. Don't delay reperfusion.
- Beta blockers
- Clopidogrel
- Heparin (UFH or LMWH)

7

Time from onset of symptoms ≤12 hours?

> 12 hours

≤ 12 hours

8

Reperfusion strategy:
Therapy defined by patient and center criteria.
- Be aware of reperfusion goals:
  – door-to-balloon inflation (PCI) goal of 90 minutes
  – door-to-needle (fibrinolysis) goal of 30 minutes
- Continue adjunctive therapies and:
  – angiotensin-converting enzyme (ACE) inhibitors/angiotensin receptor blockers (ARB) within 24 hours symptoms onset
  – HMG CoA reductase inhibitor (statin therapy).

Reproduced with permission, 2005 American Heart Association Guidelines for Cardiopulmonary Resuscitation and Emergency Cardiovascular Care © 2005, American Heart Association.

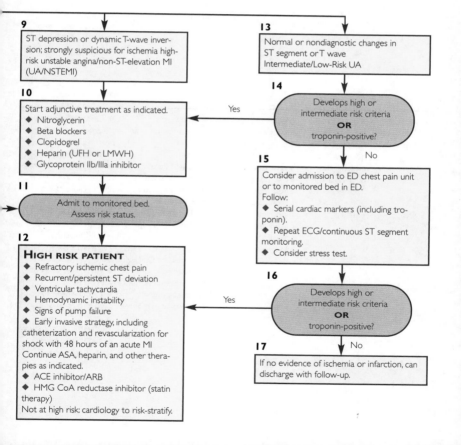

9 ST depression or dynamic T-wave inversion; strongly suspicious for ischemia high-risk unstable angina/non-ST-elevation MI (UA/NSTEMI)

10 Start adjunctive treatment as indicated.
◆ Nitroglycerin
◆ Beta blockers
◆ Clopidogrel
◆ Heparin (UFH or LMWH)
◆ Glycoprotein IIb/IIIa inhibitor

11 Admit to monitored bed. Assess risk status.

12 **HIGH RISK PATIENT**
◆ Refractory ischemic chest pain
◆ Recurrent/persistent ST deviation
◆ Ventricular tachycardia
◆ Hemodynamic instability
◆ Signs of pump failure
◆ Early invasive strategy, including catheterization and revascularization for shock with 48 hours of an acute MI
Continue ASA, heparin, and other therapies as indicated.
◆ ACE inhibitor/ARB
◆ HMG CoA reductase inhibitor (statin therapy)
Not at high risk: cardiology to risk-stratify.

13 Normal or nondiagnostic changes in ST segment or T wave Intermediate/Low-Risk UA

14 Develops high or intermediate risk criteria **OR** troponin-positive?

Yes → (to 10)
No ↓

15 Consider admission to ED chest pain unit or to monitored bed in ED.
Follow:
◆ Serial cardiac markers (including troponin).
◆ Repeat ECG/continuous ST segment monitoring.
◆ Consider stress test.

16 Develops high or intermediate risk criteria **OR** troponin-positive?

Yes → (to 12)
No ↓

17 If no evidence of ischemia or infarction, can discharge with follow-up.

CARDIAC DRUG OVERVIEW

◆

Drug	Action	Indications	Adverse Effects	Special Considerations
adenosine (Adenocard)	◆ Slows conduction through the atrioventricular (AV) node	Paroxysmal supraventricular tachycardia (PSVT)	◆ Chest pain ◆ Dyspnea ◆ Flushing ◆ Transient sinus bradycardia and ventricular ectopy	◆ Monitor cardiac rate and rhythm. ◆ A brief period of asystole (up to 15 seconds) may occur after rapid administration. ◆ Rapidly follow each dose with a 20-ml saline flush. ◆ Don't administer through a central line because a more prolonged asystole may result.
amiodarone (Cordarone)	◆ Blocks sodium channels at rapid pacing frequencies and prolongs the duration and refractory period of the action potential	Life-threatening ventricular arrhythmias, such as recurrent ventricular fibrillation and recurrent, unstable ventricular tachycardia; may be used to control rate in supraventricular arrhythmias, particularly, atrial fibrillation, and atrial flutter	◆ Bradycardia ◆ Exacerbation of arrhythmia ◆ Fever ◆ Heart failure ◆ Hepatotoxicity ◆ Hyperthyroidism ◆ Hypotension ◆ Hypothyroidism ◆ Nausea and vomiting ◆ Ophthalmic abnormalities: Corneal microdeposits ◆ Photosensitivity and skin discoloration ◆ Pulmonary fibrosis	◆ Closely monitor the patient during loading phase. ◆ If the patient needs a dosage adjustment, monitor him for an extended time because of the drug's long and variable half-life and the difficulty in predicting the time needed to achieve new steady-state plasma drug level. ◆ Administer oral doses with meals. ◆ Monitor need to adjust dose of digoxin or warfarin. ◆ Monitor pulmonary, liver, and thyroid function tests.

DRUG	ACTION	INDICATIONS	ADVERSE EFFECTS	SPECIAL CONSIDERATIONS
atropine	◆ Blocks vagal effects on the sinoatrial (SA) and AV nodes and enhances conduction through the AV node and increases the heart rate	Symptomatic sinus bradycardia, AV block, asystole and bradycardic pulseless electrical activity (PEA)	◆ Blurred vision ◆ Dry mouth ◆ Palpitations ◆ Restlessness ◆ Tachycardia ◆ Urine retention	◆ Monitor cardiac rate and rhythm. ◆ Use with caution with myocardial ischemia. ◆ Not recommended for third-degree AV block and infranodal type II second-degree AV block. ◆ In adults, avoid doses less than 0.5 mg because of risk of paradoxical slowing. ◆ Isn't effective in denervated transplanted hearts.
digoxin	◆ Increases force and velocity of myocardial contraction; slows conduction through SA and AV nodes	Slows heart rate in sinus tachycardia from heart failure and controls rapid ventricular rate in patients with atrial fibrillation or flutter	◆ AV block ◆ Bradycardia ◆ Headaches ◆ Hypokalemia ◆ Nausea and vomiting ◆ Vision disturbances	◆ Digoxin is extremely toxic, with a narrow margin of safety between therapeutic range and toxicity. ◆ Vomiting is usually an early sign of drug toxicity. ◆ Check apical pulse before giving drug and discontinue digoxin, as ordered, if patient's pulse rate falls below 60 beats/minute.
diltiazem (Cardizem)	◆ Inhibits influx of calcium through the cell membrane, resulting in a depression of automaticity and conduction velocity in smooth and cardiac muscles ◆ Different degrees of selectivity on vascular smooth muscle, myocardium, and conduction and pacemaker tissues	Atrial fibrillation, atrial flutter, atrial tachycardia	◆ Abdominal discomfort ◆ Acute hepatic injury ◆ AV block ◆ Bradycardia ◆ Dizziness ◆ Edema ◆ Headache ◆ Heart failure	◆ Closely monitor the patient when starting therapy and during dosage adjustments. ◆ May worsen heart failure. ◆ Abrupt withdrawal may result in increased frequency and duration of chest pain. ◆ Monitor cardiac and respiratory function. ◆ Don't use for a patient with Wolff-Parkinson-White (WPW) syndrome or wide-QRS tachycardia of uncertain origin. ◆ Concurrent I.V. administration with I.V. beta-adrenergic blocker may cause severe hypotension.

DRUG	ACTION	INDICATIONS	ADVERSE EFFECTS	SPECIAL CONSIDERATIONS
disopyramide (Norpace)	◆ Decreases rate of diastolic depolarization and upstroke velocity; increases action potential duration; prolongs refractory period	Life-threatening ventricular arrhythmias such as sustained ventricular tachycardia	◆ Chest pain ◆ First-degree AV block ◆ Hypotension ◆ Long QT interval ◆ Nausea ◆ Widening of QRS complex	◆ Monitor for arrhythmias and electrocardiogram (ECG) changes; notify physician of widened QRS complex or prolonged QT interval. ◆ Disopyramide increases risk of death in patients with non–life-threatening ventricular arrhythmias. ◆ Use cautiously in patients with WPW syndrome or bundle-branch block.
dofetilide (Tikosyn)	◆ Blocks cardiac potassium channels; increases duration of action potential by delaying repolarization	Maintains sinus rhythm in patients with chronic atrial fibrillation or atrial flutter	◆ Chest pain ◆ Headache ◆ Torsades de pointes	◆ Don't use if baseline QTc is greater than 440 msec, if baseline heart rate is less than 50 beats/minute, or if severe renal impairment exists. ◆ Must be initiated by cardiologist, with continuous ECG monitoring for at least 3 days. ◆ Don't use with cimetidine, verapamil, ketoconazole, or trimethoprim.
epinephrine	◆ Stimulates alpha and beta receptors in the sympathetic nervous system; relaxes bronchial smooth muscle by stimulating beta$_2$ receptors	Cardiac arrest (ventricular fibrillation [VF], pulseless ventricular tachycardia, asystole, PEA), symptomatic bradycardia, and for treatment of bronchospasm and anaphylaxis	◆ Angina ◆ Cerebral hemorrhage ◆ Hypertension ◆ Nervousness ◆ Palpitations ◆ Tachycardia	◆ Monitor cardiac rate and rhythm and blood pressure because increased heart rate and blood pressure may cause myocardial ischemia. ◆ Don't mix I.V. dose with alkaline solutions. ◆ Give drug into a large vein to prevent irritation or extravasation at site.
flecainide (Tambocor)	◆ Decreases excitability, conduction velocity and automaticity due to slowed atrial, AV node, His-Purkinje system, and intraventricular conduction	Ventricular arrhythmias, supraventricular arrhythmias (patients without coronary artery disease), and atrial fibrillation and atrial flutter	◆ Dizziness ◆ Dyspnea ◆ Headache ◆ Nausea ◆ Ventricular arrhythmias (new or worsened) ◆ Vision disturbances	◆ Contraindicated in patients with impaired left-ventricular function. ◆ Periodically monitor trough plasma levels because 40% is bound to plasma protein. ◆ Increase dosage as ordered at intervals of more than 4 days in patients with renal disease.

DRUG	ACTION	INDICATIONS	ADVERSE EFFECTS	SPECIAL CONSIDERATIONS
flecainide (continued)				◆ Monitor for ECG changes, prolonged PR interval, widening QRS complex, and lengthening of QT interval.
ibutilide (Corvert)	◆ Delays repolarization by activating slow, inward current (mostly sodium), which results in prolonged duration of atrial and ventricular action potential and refractoriness	Rapid conversion of recent-onset atrial fibrillation or atrial flutter	◆ Headache ◆ Hypotension ◆ Nausea ◆ Prolonged QT interval ◆ Torsades de pointes ◆ Worsening ventricular tachycardia	◆ Stop drug infusion as ordered when arrhythmia stops, if ventricular tachycardia occurs, or if QT interval becomes markedly prolonged. ◆ Perform continuous ECG monitoring for at least 4 hours after dose is completed because of proarrhythmic risk. ◆ Check potassium and magnesium levels and correct before giving drug.
lidocaine (Xylocaine)	◆ Shortens the refractory period and suppresses the automaticity of ectopic foci without affecting conduction of impulses through cardiac tissue	Acute ventricular arrhythmias, such as ventricular tachycardia and VF	◆ Dizziness ◆ Hallucinations ◆ Nervousness ◆ Seizures ◆ Tachycardia ◆ Tachypnea	◆ Monitor cardiac rhythm and notify physician of prolonged PR interval and widened QRS complex. ◆ Contraindicated in second- or third-degree AV block without pacing support, WPW syndrome, and Stokes-Adams syndrome. ◆ Reduce drug dosage as ordered in patients with heart failure or liver disease. ◆ Monitor patient closely for central nervous system changes.
moricizine (Ethmozine)	◆ Shortens phase II and III repolarization, leading to decreased duration of the action potential and an effective refractory period	Life-threatening ventricular arrhythmias such as sustained ventricular tachycardia	◆ Bradycardia ◆ Dizziness ◆ Headache ◆ Nausea ◆ Sustained ventricular tachycardia	◆ Use cautiously in patients with sick sinus syndrome because of the possibility of sinus arrest. ◆ The patient should be hospitalized for initial dosing and monitored for heart failure. ◆ Give before meals because food delays rate of absorption.

DRUG	ACTION	INDICATIONS	ADVERSE EFFECTS	SPECIAL CONSIDERATIONS
procainamide (Procanbid, Pronestyl)	◆ Produces a direct cardiac effect to prolong the refractory period of the atria and (to a lesser extent) the His-Purkinje system and the ventricles	Potentially life-threatening ventricular arrhythmias; and atrial fibrillation with rapid rate in WPW syndrome	◆ Agranulocytosis ◆ Diarrhea ◆ Dizziness ◆ Heart block ◆ Hypotension ◆ Liver failure ◆ Lupus erythematosus-like syndrome ◆ Nausea and vomiting	◆ Monitor for arrhythmias and notify physician of widened QRS complex or prolonged QT interval. ◆ Procainamide increases risk of death in patients with non–life-threatening arrhythmias. ◆ Use with caution in patients with liver or kidney dysfunction. ◆ Tell patient not to crush or break extended-release tablets.
propafenone (Rythmol)	◆ Reduces upstroke velocity of monophasic action potential ◆ Reduces fast, inward current carried by sodium ions in Purkinje fibers ◆ Increases diastolic excitability threshold ◆ Prolongs effective refractory period	Life-threatening ventricular arrhythmias such as ventricular tachycardia when benefits of treatment outweigh risks	◆ AV block ◆ Constipation ◆ Dizziness ◆ Headache ◆ Nausea and vomiting ◆ Unusual taste ◆ Ventricular tachycardia	◆ Monitor liver and renal function studies. ◆ Report significant widening of QRS complex and evidence of second- or third-degree AV block. ◆ Increase dosage more gradually, as ordered, in elderly patients and patients with previous myocardial damage.
propranolol (Inderal)	◆ Antiarrhythmic action results from beta-adrenergic receptor blockade as well as a direct membrane stabilization action on cardiac cells	Ventricular tachycardias, supraventricular arrhythmias, and premature ventricular contractions	◆ AV block ◆ Bradycardia ◆ Bronchospasm ◆ Heart failure ◆ Hypotension ◆ Light-headedness ◆ Nausea and vomiting	◆ Propranolol is also used for treatment of hypertension, angina pectoris, and myocardial infarction (MI). ◆ Dosages may differ for hypertension, angina, or MI. ◆ Check apical pulse before giving drug. If extremes in pulse rate occur, stop drug and notify practitioner immediately. ◆ Report significant lengthening of PR interval and monitor for AV block. ◆ Drug masks common signs and symptoms of shock and hypoglycemia. ◆ Use cautiously in patients with reactive airway disease (asthma).

DRUG	ACTION	INDICATIONS	ADVERSE EFFECTS	SPECIAL CONSIDERATIONS
sotalol (Betapace)	◆ Antiarrhythmic with beta-blocking effects and prolongation of the action potential ◆ Slows AV nodal conduction and increases AV nodal refractoriness	Life-threatening ventricular arrhythmias; maintains sinus rhythm in patients with history of symptomatic atrial fibrillation or atrial flutter	◆ Bradycardia ◆ Chest pain ◆ Dizziness ◆ Fatigue ◆ Palpitations ◆ QT prolongation	◆ Contraindicated in patients with bronchial asthma, sinus bradycardia, or second- or third-degree AV block without a pacemaker. ◆ Perform ECG monitoring for at least 3 days when therapy starts. ◆ Adjust dosage in renally impaired patients. ◆ Monitor patient for QTc prolongation. ◆ Administer drug when patient has an empty stomach.
vasopressin	◆ Antidiuretic hormone acts at the cyclic adenosine monophosphate (cAMP) and increases permeability of renal tubular epithelium to water; at high doses, is a powerful vasoconstrictor of capillaries and small arterioles and may help maintain coronary perfusion pressure	Cardiac arrest with VF as an alternative to epinephrine	◆ Bronchoconstriction ◆ Chest pain ◆ Hypersensitivity ◆ Myocardial ischemia ◆ Water intoxication	◆ Monitor cardiac rhythm and blood pressure. ◆ Assess for hypersensitivity reactions, including urticaria, angioedema, bronchoconstriction, and anaphylaxis.

SELECTED REFERENCES

"AHA Scientific Statement: Practice Standards for Electrocardiographic Monitoring in Hospital Setting," *Circulation* 110(17):2721-46, October 2004.

Albert, N.M. "Cardiac Resynchronization Therapy through Biventricular Pacing in Patients with Heart Failure and Ventricular Dyssynchrony," *Critical Care Nurse* 23(3 Suppl):2-13, June 2003.

ECG Interpretation Made Incredibly Easy, 3rd ed. Philadelphia: Lippincott Williams & Wilkins, 2005.

Fuster, V., et al., eds. *Atherothrombosis and Coronary Artery Disease,* 2nd ed. Philadelphia: Lippincott Williams & Wilkins, 2005.

Geiter, H. "Critical Care: Getting Back to Basics with Permanent Pacemakers, Part II," *Nursing* 34(11):32cc1-32cc2, November 2004.

Handbook of Emergency Cardiovascular Care for Healthcare Providers. Dallas: American Heart Association, 2006.

Interpreting Difficult ECGs: A Rapid Reference. Philadelphia: Lippincott Williams & Wilkins, 2006.

LeRoy, S.S. "Long QT syndrome and Other Repolarization-related Dysrhythmias," *AACN Clinical Issues Advanced Practice in Acute and Critical Care: Electrophysiology and Device Therapy* 15(3):419-431, July-September, 2004.

Mastering ACLS, 2nd ed. Philadelphia: Lippincott Williams & Wilkins, 2006.

Morton, S., et al. *Critical Care Nursing: A Holistic Approach,* 8th ed. Philadelphia: Lippincott Williams & Wilkins, 2005.

Nursing2007 Drug Handbook, 27th ed. Philadelphia: Lippincott Williams & Wilkins, 2007.

Pyne, C.C. "Classification of Acute Coronary Syndromes Using the 12-lead Electrocardiogram as a Guide," *AACN Clinical Issues Advanced Practice in Acute and Critical Care: Advanced Assessment* 15(4):558-567, October-December, 2004.

Shea, J.B. "Quality of Life Issues in Patients with Implantable Cardioverter Defibrillators Driving, Occupation and Recreation," *AACN Clinical Issues Advanced Practice in Acute and Critical Care: Electrophysiology and Device Therapy* 15(3):478-489, July-September, 2004.

Skillmasters Expert ECG Interpretation, 2nd ed. Philadelphia: Lippincott Williams & Wilkins, 2007.

Thompson, E., et al. "Radiofrequency Ablation in the Pulmonary Veins for Paroxysmal, Drug-resistant Atrial Fibrillation," *Dimensions of Critical Care Nursing* 23(6):255-263, November-December 2004.

Woods, S.L., et al. *Cardiac Nursing,* 5th ed. Philadelphia: Lippincott Williams & Wilkins, 2005.

INDEX

---

i refers to an illustration; t refers to a table.

i refers to an illustration; t refers to a table.

Electrical axis *(continued)*
quadrant method for determination of, 148-149, 150i
on 12-lead electrocardiogram, 135-137
Electrical impulse transmission, 12-13
abnormal, 19, 82, 85
in bundle-branch block, 168
cardiac conduction system, 16-19, 16i
depolarization-repolarization cycle, 13-16, 14t
in Wolff-Parkinson-White syndrome, 83i
Electrical interference, 45, 45t
Electrocardiogram, 16, 20-37
artifacts on, 44-45t, 45-46
Ashman's phenomenon on, 79i
cardiac drug effects on, 187-193, 188-193i
current direction and waveform deflection on, 21, 21i
8-step method for analyzing rhythm strip, 33-37, 34i
electrode placement, 22-25, 23i, 40-41i
examining electrocardiogram grid, 25, 26i
leads, 20-26, 23i
pacemaker spike on, 194-195, 195i
planes, 21
practice strips for interpretation of, 225-250
12-lead, 22, 135-143, 144-146i. *See also* 12-lead electrocardiogram.
waveform components of, 26-32, 27-32i
Electrocardiogram monitoring, 38-46
application of electrodes for, 39, 40i, 42-43
dual-lead, 39, 41i
EASI system, 39, 42i
hardwire, 38
leadwire systems for, 39-43, 40-42i
observing cardiac rhythm, 43
telemetry, 38, 40-41i

Electrocardiogram monitoring *(continued)*
troubleshooting monitor problems, 44-45t, 45-46
Electrodes, electrocardiogram
application of, 39, 42-43
placement of, 22-25, 23i, 40-41i
for 12-lead electrocardiogram, 137-141, 138-140i
Electrodes, pacemaker, 195
Electrolyte disturbances, 125-131
Electromagnetic interference, 211
Endocardium, 4, 5i
Enlargement, atrial, 177, 178-179, 178i, 179i
Epicardial pacemaker, 203
Epicardium, 4, 5i
Epinephrine, 270t
Esmolol, 190
Ethmozine. *See* Moricizine.
Excitability of cardiac cells, 12-13

FG

Failure to capture as pacemaker problem, 206, 207i
Failure to pace as pacemaker problem, 206-208, 207i
Fascicular block, 172-177
left anterior, 168, 172-174, 174i, 175i
left posterior, 168, 174-176, 176i, 177i
trifascicular, 176-177
Fast channel blockers, 187
Fibrillation waves, 73, 74i
1,500 method of heart rate calculation, 35
First-degree atrioventricular block, 115-117
causes of, 116
clinical significance of, 116
electrocardiogram characteristics of, 115, 116i, 258i
interventions for, 117
signs and symptoms of, 117
treatment of, 117
Five-leadwire system, 39, 40-41i
Flecainide, 188, 270-271t

Flutter waves, 70, 71i
F waves, 70, 71i, 73

H

Hardwire monitoring, 38-43, 40-41i
Heart
autonomic innervation of, 12
blood flow through, 7-8
blood supply to, 8-10, 9i
chambers of, 5-6
electrical conduction system of, 16-19, 16i
location of, 3, 4i
physiology of, 10-19
structure of, 3-4, 7i
valves of, 6-7, 7i
wall of, 4, 5i
Heart murmur, 6
Heart rate calculation, 35, 36t
Hemiblock. *See* Fascicular block.
Hexaxial reference system, 148, 149i
Hypercalcemia, 128-130
causes of, 129
clinical significance of, 129
electrocardiogram characteristics of, 129, 129i
interventions for, 129-130
signs and symptoms of, 129
Hyperkalemia, 125-127
causes of, 125-126
clinical significance of, 126
electrocardiogram characteristics of, 126, 126i
interventions for, 126-127
signs and symptoms of, 126
Hypertrophy, ventricular, 177-178, 179-181, 180i, 181i
Hypocalcemia, 130-131
causes of, 130
clinical significance of, 130
electrocardiogram characteristics of, 130, 131i
interventions for, 131
signs and symptoms of, 130
Hypokalemia, 127-128
causes of, 127
clinical significance of, 127
electrocardiogram characteristics of, 127-128, 128i
interventions for, 128

i refers to an illustration; t refers to a table.

i refers to an illustration; t refers to a table.

Moricizine, 188, 271t
Multifocal atrial tachycardia, 66, 67i, 69. *See also* Atrial tachycardia.
  distinguishing from atrial fibrillation, 75, 77i, 245i
Myocardial infarction, 152
  anterior wall, 163t, 164i
  distinguishing from acute pericarditis, 160i
  electrocardiogram characteristics of, 152, 155-158, 160i, 164-167i
  inferior wall, 165, 166i
  interventions for, 158-162
  lateral wall, 165, 165i
  locating myocardial damage in, 162, 163t
  posterior wall, 165-167
  release of cardiac enzymes and proteins in, 158, 162
  right ventricular, 167, 167i
  septal wall, 163-164
  signs and symptoms of, 154
  stages of myocardial ischemia, injury and, 159i
Myocardium, 4, 5i, 7i
  contractility of, 12

N
Nonpharmacologic treatments, 194-221
Normal sinus rhythm, 32-37, 33i, 34i
  risk of restoring in atrial fibrillation, 75
Norpace. *See* Disopyramide.

O
Overdrive suppression, 68-69
Oversensing as pacemaker problem, 208

P
Pacemaker cells, 12, 17, 19. *See also* Sinoatrial node.
  action potential curves for, 15i
  ectopic, in ventricles, 96
  junctional, 82, 84-85
Pacemakers, 194-212
  for asynchronous pacing, 196
  components of, 194-195, 195i

Pacemakers *(continued)*
  description codes for, 196, 197
  distinguishing intermittent ventricular pacing from premature ventricular contractions, 206i, 250i
  electrocardiogram effects of, 194-195, 195i
  electromagnetic interference with, 211
  evaluating function of, 205, 210
  indications for, 194
  modes of, 196-200, 198-200i
  permanent, 200-202
    biventricular, 200-202, 202i, 209, 212
    interventions for patients with, 209
    placement of, 201i
    teaching patients about, 211-212
  programming of, 196-200
  for synchronous pacing, 196
  temporary, 194, 202-205
    epicardial, 203
    interventions for patients with, 210-211
    pulse generator for, 204i
    settings for, 204-205
    teaching patients about, 212
    transcutaneous, 100, 100i, 203
    transthoracic, 204
    transvenous, 203
  troubleshooting problems with, 205-208, 207-208i
PACs. *See* Premature atrial contractions.
Paper-and-pencil method of measuring rhythm, 34i
Papillary muscles, 6, 7i
Paroxysmal atrial tachycardia, 66, 67i, 68, 69. *See also* Atrial tachycardia.
Pericardial fluid, 5
Pericardial space, 5
Pericarditis, 152
  distinguishing from myocardial infarction, 160i
  electrocardiogram characteristics of, 160i, 161i
Pericardium, 4-5, 5i

Pharmacologic treatments, 185-193, 268-273t
Phenytoin, 188
PJCs. *See* Premature junctional contractions.
Planes, 21
Posterior-lead electrocardiogram, 141, 142i
Potassium, 13-14, 14t, 125. *See also* Hyperkalemia; Hypokalemia.
Potassium channel blockers, 191, 191i
PR interval, 28-29, 28i, 33, 33i
  determining duration of, 37
Precordial leads, 24-25, 135, 136t, 140-141, 140i
  placement of, 140-141, 140i
  views reflected by, 135, 136i
Preexcitation syndromes, 83i
Preload, 12, 13i
Premature atrial contractions, 63-65
  causes of, 63
  clinical significance of, 63
  conducted, 63
  distinguishing from wandering pacemaker, 80, 81i, 246i
  electrocardiogram characteristics of, 64i, 65i, 81i, 121i, 254i
  interventions for, 64-65
  nonconducted, 63
    distinguishing from sinoatrial block, 63, 65, 65i
    distinguishing from type II second-degree atrioventricular block, 120, 121i, 249i
  signs and symptoms of, 63-64
  treatment of, 64
Premature junctional contractions, 83-84
  causes of, 83-84
  clinical significance of, 84
  electrocardiogram characteristics of, 85i, 256i
  interventions for, 84
  signs and symptoms of, 84
  treatment of, 84

---

i refers to an illustration; t refers to a table.

Premature ventricular contractions, 92-96
in bigeminy or trigeminy, 93, 95i
causes of, 94
clinical significance of, 94
distinguishing from intermittent ventricular pacing, 206i, 250i
distinguishing from ventricular aberrancy, 96, 97i
electrocardiogram characteristics of, 92-93, 93i, 95i, 97i, 206i, 257i
interventions for, 96
multiform, 93, 95i
paired, 92, 95i
in R-on-T phenomenon, 95i
signs and symptoms of, 95, 96
treatment of, 96
unifocal versus multifocal, 94
Prinzmetal angina, 153-154
Procainamide, 187, 272t
Procanbid. See Procainamide.
Pronestyl. See Procainamide.
Propafenone, 188, 272t
Propranolol, 190, 272t
Pulmonary arteries, 6, 7i
Pulmonary circulation, 7
Pulmonary embolism, 55
Pulmonary veins, 5, 7, 7i
ablation of, 217, 218i
Pulmonic valve, 6, 7i
Pulseless arrest, advanced cardiac life support algorithm for, 260-261i
Pulseless electrical activity, 113
Purkinje fibers, 16i, 18-19
PVCs. See Premature ventricular contractions.
P wave, 26-28, 27i, 33, 33i
evaluation of, 35
in junctional arrhythmias, 82, 84i
variations of, 28, 28i

Q

QRS complex, 29-30, 30i, 33, 33i, 168
determining duration of, 37
QT interval, 31-32, 32i, 33, 33i
determining duration of, 37

Quadrant method for determining electrical axis, 148-149, 150i
Quinidine, 187

R

Radiofrequency ablation, 69, 217-219
indications for, 217
patient interventions after, 219
procedure for, 217, 218i
teaching patient about, 219
Rapid atrial pacing, 68-69
RBBB. See Right bundle-branch block.
Reentry, 18i, 19, 62
Repolarization, 13-16, 14t
Resting potential, 13
Retrograde conduction, 19, 82, 85
Rhythm strip, 22, 142-143
8-step method for analyzing, 33-37, 34i
labeling of, 43, 143
observing cardiac rhythm on, 43
practice strips for interpretation of, 225-250
Right atrial enlargement, 178
causes of, 178
electrocardiogram characteristics of, 178, 178i
interventions for, 178
signs and symptoms of, 178
Right bundle-branch aberrancy, 97i
Right bundle-branch block, 168, 169
causes of, 169
electrocardiogram characteristics of, 169, 171i
interventions for, 169
signs and symptoms of, 169
understanding, 169, 170i
Right chest–lead electrocardiogram, 141, 143i
Right ventricular hypertrophy, 179-180
causes of, 179
electrocardiogram characteristics of, 179-180, 180i
interventions for, 180
signs and symptoms of, 180
R-on-T phenomenon, 95i

R-R interval, 32
Rythmol. See Propafenone.

S

Second-degree atrioventricular block, 117-121
type I, 117-118
type II, 119-121
Semilunar valves, 6-7, 7i
Sequence method of heart rate calculation, 35
Sick sinus syndrome, 58-61
causes of, 59-60
clinical significance of, 60
electrocardiogram characteristics of, 59i
interventions for, 61
signs and symptoms of, 60-61
treatment of, 61
Sinoatrial exit block, 55-58
causes of, 56-57
clinical significance of, 57-58
differentiation from sinus arrest, 58
distinguishing from premature atrial contractions, 63, 65, 65i
electrocardiogram characteristics of, 57i, 65i
interventions for, 58
signs and symptoms of, 58
treatment of, 58
Sinoatrial node, 4, 16i, 17, 49
Sinoatrial node arrhythmias, 49-61
Sinoatrial syndrome. See Sick sinus syndrome.
Sinus arrest, 55-58
causes of, 56-57
clinical significance of, 57-58
differentiation from SA exit block, 58
electrocardiogram characteristics of, 55, 56i, 254i
interventions for, 58
signs and symptoms of, 58
treatment of, 58
Sinus arrhythmia, 49-51
causes of, 49-50
clinical significance of, 50
electrocardiogram characteristics of, 50, 50i, 253i
interventions for, 51
signs and symptoms of, 50
treatment of, 50-51

---

i refers to an illustration; t refers to a table.

i refers to an illustration; t refers to a table.